REMOVE THE "SPLINTERS" AND WATCH THE BODY HEAL

Defining the Real Cause of "disease" and How to Fix It Naturally

DR. GERALD H. SMITH

Digitally produced in the United States of America

Remove the "Splinters" and Watch the Body Heal
Defining the Real Cause of "Disease" and How To Fix It Naturally

Author: **Dr. Gerald H. Smith**

Editing by: **Evelyn Adler and Dr. Gerald H. Smith**

Front cover duck image: **Ashley Saunders**

Front cover design: **Johanna Bellerose**

All case photographs and videos taken by: **Dr. Gerald H. Smith**

Main category: **Health**

First Edition

Publisher: **International Center For Nutritional Research, Inc.**

303 Corporate Drive East • Langhorne, PA 19047

Web site: **www.icnr.com**

Table of Contents

a. Child's Seizures Followed Four Month Schedule of Vaccines How Safe is Your Child's Vaccine?

b. Why Corporate Medicine is a Poor Investment

c. The Mystery of Bipolar Disorder Solved

d. Symptoms of Mercury Toxicity

e. Eight Years of Chronic Pain Due to Third Molar Extractions

f. What is Cranial Manipulation and Why is it so Important?

g. Twenty-one Years and Nine Months Post Concussion Symptoms Resolved in One Treatment

h. Twenty Years of Migraine Headaches Resolved with One Cranial Adjustment

i. Post-Whiplash Sequelae of Eight Months Resolved in OneTreatment

j. One and a Half Years Post-Whiplash Pain Resolved

k. Post-Whiplash Pain

l. Fifteen Year Migraine Headaches Resolved

m. Concussion Revisited: Sixteen Years Post-Concussion Syndrome Resolved in One and a Half Hours

Preface

Remove The "Splinters" and Watch the Body Heal was written to fill a void in our present healthcare system. The concepts put forth in this book will help guide practitioners back to the basics of healing, rekindle the need for common sense, and define how to take a logical approach to evaluating patients' symptoms and how to utilize appropriate treatment modalities. Medical technology has become so sophisticated that physicians and patients alike have become paralyzed by over-analysis and have lost sight of how the body really works. A comprehensive diagnostic and treatment system is offered here to approach the patient's problems from a global perspective rather than just to treat his or her symptoms. My intention is to instill the philosophy of less is more and to show that the closer one gets to the truth, the more simplistic the solution.

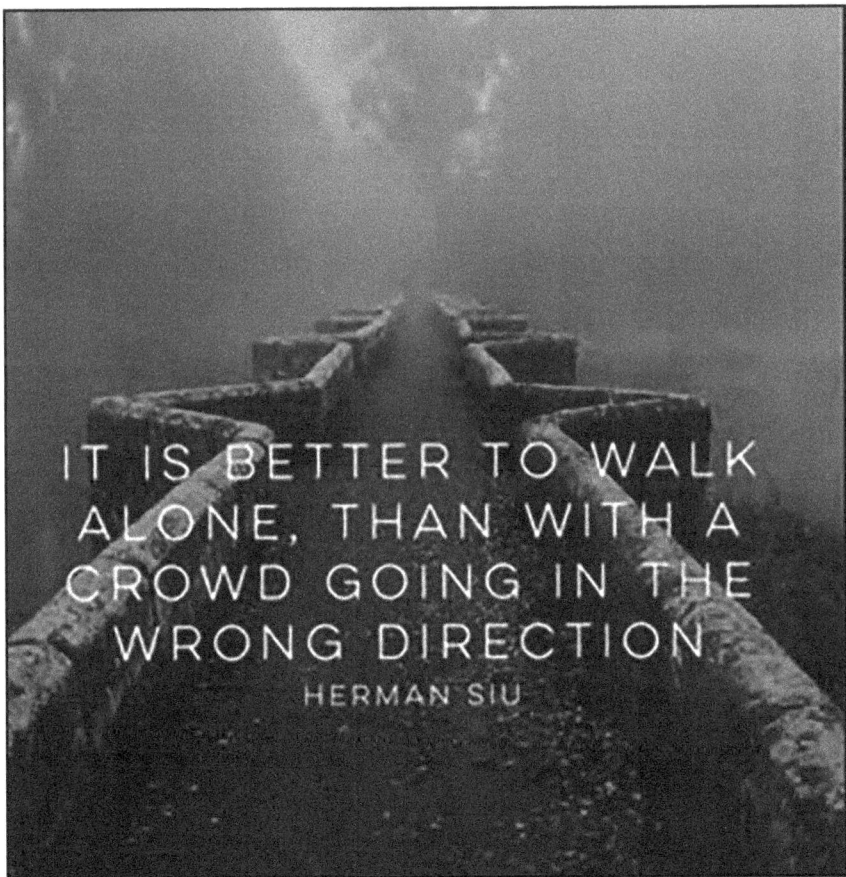

IT IS BETTER TO WALK ALONE, THAN WITH A CROWD GOING IN THE WRONG DIRECTION
HERMAN SIU

Biography

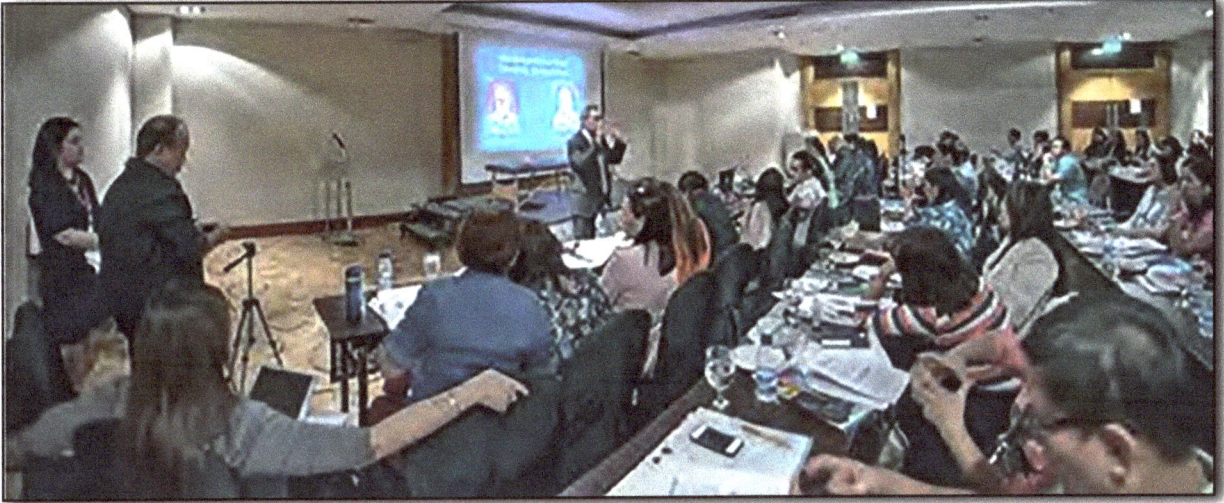

Doctor Smith Presenting A Lecture in Manila

Doctor Smith graduated Temple School of Dentistry in 1969 and completed a two-year tour of active duty as a captain in the U.S. Army Dental Corp. After practicing conventional dentistry for four years, Dr. Smith completed a two-year post-graduate orthodontic program in 1976. Sir, Doctor Smith is a Knight Hospitaller a dedicated professional organization dating back to the year 1050. The Knights Hospitallers have official recognition from the United Nations and the Pope for there tremendous humanitarian work with the poor. Doctor Smith is certified by the World Organization For Natural Medicine to practice natural medicine.

Dr. Smith's broad base of post-graduate training has enabled him to integrate many health care specialties. He has accumulated an impressive list of credentials, which includes lecturing at Walter Reed Army Medical Center, National Academy of General Dentistry, Academy of Head, Neck and Facial Pain, Yonsei Memorial Hospital in Seoul Korea and dozens of guest lecture appearances at national and international symposia. He holds memberships and affiliations with a number of professional associations including the International Associations for Orthodontists and Academy of Head, Neck and Facial Pain. He has been an active member of the Holistic Dental Association since 1993, past-president of the Holistic Dental

Biography

Association and editor of their professional journal from 2003 to 2006. He also served as past-president of the Pennsylvania Craniomandibular Society.

Dr. Smith is a recognized international authority and pioneer in craniomandibular somatic disorders with a focus on resolving chronic pain. Dr. Smith was the first researcher in the world to document cranial bone motion by means of his ground breaking research and development of the Dental Orthogonal Radiographic Analysis System. He was also the first researcher in the world to discover how to resolve chronic pain by removing tension patterns within the human skull by means of the Occlusal Cranial Balancing Technique. He is author of two landmark textbooks for professionals, Cranial-Dental-Sacral Complex and Dental Orthogonal Radiographic Analysis. He has also written an important book for the lay person, Headaches Aren't Forever, a downloadable E-book, Alternative Treatments For Conquering Chronic Pain, and Reversing Cancer: A Journey From Cancer to Cure — a survivors guide for understanding the nature of cancer, restoring the immune system, psychological healing, destroying cancer, and regeneration. Doctor Smith's fifty years of clinical research has identified several of the major missing links for successfully treating dentally related medical issues, cancer, and chronic pain.

In addition, Dr. Smith has published over thirty articles and contributed chapters to several professional books, developer of the Physiologic Adaptive Range Concept, Occlusal Cranial Balancing Technique, Quantum Testing Technique and a special dental x-ray analysis system for measuring cranial bone motion. He holds two US Patents: a unique precision attachment for dental fixed bridgework and second patent for a flash adaptor to facilitate taking intraoral photographs. Doctor Smith is also president of the International Center For Nutritional Research, Inc. and he still maintains a private practice in Bucks County Pennsylvania, where he focuses his integrative healing concepts on chronic pain patients.

Remove the "Splinters" and Watch the Body Heal

Introduction

The motivation to write this book was simple. Both my parents and my wife were killed by the technologies of "modern medicine." In addition, when I was just a ten month-old baby the medical establishment put the fear of God into my parents and convinced them that they had to irradiate my enlarged thymus gland to prevent me from possibly chocking to death. In the process, they destroyed part of my thyroid gland. In hindsight, it is amazing that I made it through four years of undergraduate school and four years of professional school. I literally had to study five times harder than the other students to remember anything.

In a world where Big Pharma controls the media and the dissemination of false information is rampant, it is my hope that putting out my fifty years of clinical research on how the body really works will open the eyes and minds of the average citizen and physicians. The public has been led to believe that natural medicine is an alternative and not a traditional or mainstream treatment and that pharmaceutical drugs, which came on the scene in the late 1940's, represents conventional or traditional medicine — the one and only way to go. It is amazing how mind control techniques and an overload of statistics can brainwash the public into believing that chemical drugs represent traditional medicine when in fact herbs, homeopathic medicines, vitamins, and healing with light and magnetic fields were on the scene long before pharmaceutical drugs were discovered.

Current science-based medicine provides state-of-the-art diagnostic technology with one major exception: the inability to diagnose the real underlying causative factors of disease. Once the public realizes that traditional medical testing, in particular, blood tests, only reveal reactions to the underlying cause and not the actual cause, people will gravitate to systems that use vibrational analysis for their diagnostic answers. A case in point was one of my patients, Fred S., who suffered from a swollen liver for twenty-seven years. The medical establishment recommended that Fred undergo a liver transplant, which he refused. All the fancy blood analysis and modern diagnostic testing could not reveal the underlying cause of the problem. In one hour, using energy testing, it was revealed that Fred had benzene and hepatitis B in his liver. After seven months on a nutritional program to remove the two offending "splinters", Fred's liver went back to normal and so did his liver enzymes. This scenario occurred in 2011, and Fred has been living the good life ever since with his own liver.

The paradigm that is being introduced in this book is based on quantum physics. Since the entire universe is made up of frequencies, all abnormalities have a signature frequency by which they can be determined. Sophisticated diagnostic software exists which is noninvasive, accurate, and cost-effective and available to the average patient. The missing key in the health equation is the enlightenment of the patient and the denial of the medical community. As Albert Einstein once stated, "The mind, once stretched by a new idea, never returns to its original dimensions." Once people wake up to the truth and embrace reality, they will reject pharmaceutical based "traditional medicine."

Medicine in the Twenty-First Century

The New Millennium has ushered in a major paradigm shift in medicine: define and treat the underlying cause. Based on concepts of quantum physics and an integration of many specialities this unique therapy is called Quantum Medicine. Based on intelligent evolution[1], patented technologies, and outside the box innovative thinking a more comprehensive evaluation and treatment approach now exists. Enlightened practitioners now look at the patient globally and incorporate factors which traditional medicine reject, discount or are not even aware. Innovative technologies focus on reciprocal structural issues (skull bone distortions which can affect the entire spinal nerves and vertebrae alignment), Dental problems (toxic root canal teeth, jawbone infections, mercury fillings, malocclusions, galvanic currents among dissimilar metals in the mouth, incompatible and toxic dental materials, faulty orthodontics all of which can affect the entire body), spinal/pelvic misalignments, soft tissue abnormalities (fascial distortions, muscle imbalances, lymphatic drainage issues), toxic effects of vaccines (Tetanus, MMR, Gardasil, flu shots, etc.) emotional issues (imprinted during pregnancy, childhood and adulthood can be the root cause of chronic pain and/or structural imbalances), stealth organisms (cytomegalovirus, Mycoplasma fermentans, Lyme disease, MRSA, Chemtrail toxins, etc.), radiation from Fukushima, Japan, trapped medications (antibiotics, vaccines, statins, anti-nausea drugs like Bendectin and thalidomide) in various organs and tissues, and the dangerous effects of microwaves (smart meters, cell phones, and wi-fi) which are associated with causing cancers, Parkinson's disease, Alzheimer's, chronic fatigue, insomnia and depression and have been implicated in re-initiating such diseases after they have been placed in remission. Unless more patients become enlightened and start demanding these advanced evaluations and treatments, the patient's quality of life will continue to be denied due to ignorance. The following cliff note versions of case studies have been presented to drive home the power of Quantum Medicine. Patients now have a choice: treat your symptoms with science based medicine and hope for the best or seek out noninvasive Quantum Medicine and treat the underlying cause and effect a cure.

Case 1. Chronic Itching and Wheat-Gluten Sensitivity

A six year-old child was referred for the chief complaint of constant scratching and sensitivity to foods with wheat and gluten. After a comprehensive evaluation, the child was diagnosed with Tetanus vaccine trapped in the left lobe of her thyroid gland. After two days on a homeopathic remedy, the child's itching dramatically reduced allowing her to sleep through the night, which she was unable to do for several years. Another side effect of neutralizing the trapped Tetanus vaccine was that she was able to tolerate wheat and gluten without breaking out in a rash.

Case 2. Enlarged Liver for 27 Years

Fred was brought to my office with the chief complaint of having a swollen liver for 27 years. In addition to his jaundiced appearance, Fred lost his zest for life, and he would lose his train of thought in the middle of a sentence. Conventional medicine's solution to Fred's problem was to do a liver transplant, which he refused. Following a comprehensive examination with the newer Quantum Testing technologies, Fred was diagnosed with hepatitis B and benzene in his liver. After 7 months of treatment with natural remedies to remove the two causative factors, Fred's liver totally went back to normal. His pre-treatment blood tests showed a high reading for alkaline phosphatase (reflects elevated liver enzymes), which went back to normal.

Case 3. Patient was Going Blind in Her Left Eye

Pat was referred to my practice for the chief complaint of going blind in her left eye. Pat was being treated by a world class hospital where the physician was injecting her eye with a chemotherapeutic drug, Avastin, which cuts the blood supply to tumors. A comprehensive evaluation diagnosed cytomegalovirus in the eye. Four months of treatment with specific natural herbs, vitamins and homeopathic remedies, Pat regained full vision in the left eye. An interesting side note was the fact that the examination also revealed a low functioning thyroid gland. Nine months of therapy to correct the hypothyroid condition resulted in Pat losing 70 pounds and looks and feels ten years younger.

Case 4. Wide Spread Blisters, Itching and Burning Sensations

An eight year-old girl was referred for the presence of wide spread blisters on her arms, legs, and torso. The patient was being treated by a world class childrens hospital for the past two years with antibiotics and steroids with no success. Sixty doctors had consulted on the case and the lesions were even biopsied. All their science based medicine could not figure out the underlying cause. A complete examination with noninvasive technologies diagnosed herpes zoster (shingles), and Herpes simplex, and Candida. Four months of natural homeopathic remedies resulted in total resolution of the blisters and symptoms.

Case 5. Persistent Coughing

A four year-old male was referred for constant coughing which did not respond to conventional medicine. A noninvasive, comprehensive examination revealed Mycoplasma pneumonia, which is a common pathogen present in Chemtrail spraying across our nation. With in two days of the patient taking a Chemtrail homeopathic remedy, the coughing totally ceased.

Case 6. Stage IV Throat Cancer

A 76 year-old male was referred with a medical diagnosis of stage IV throat cancer. When the patient told his oncologist he was going for alternative treatment, the oncologist said it was a farce and waste of time and money. Of primary interest is the association of infected teeth as an interference field and supplier of pathogens for cancer. The comprehensive examination revealed two infected root canal treated teeth. The same pathogens that were present in the infected teeth were also present in the exact area of the throat cancer. The two infected teeth were extracted.

Ozone, homeopathics and ionic silver were used to treat the extraction site. The patient was placed on a raw foods diet, bio-frequency treatments and underwent Insulin Potentiation Therapy by an alternative physician. In three weeks the patient's cancer was gone. PET Scan, blood tests and visual examination by the original oncologist revealed no cancer.

Case 7. Polycythemia Vera: Serious Blood Disorder

A sixty-two year-old male physician was referred for dental evaluation in relationship to the patient's medical diagnosis of Polycythemia vera. The Mayo Clinic describes this disease as "a slow-growing type of blood cancer in which your bone marrow makes too many red blood cells. Polycythemia vera may also result in production of too many of the other types of blood cells—white blood cells and platelets. These excess cells thicken your blood and cause complications, such as a risk of blood clots or bleeding. "This rare disease is life threatening if not treated. The gold standard, science based treatment given was blood letting, every three weeks, by a very prestigious hospital. The patient had numerous mercury fillings, which give off mercury into the mouth 24/7. Treatment involved a comprehensive nutritional program to chelate out the expelled mercury and detox the liver and other tissues. Following the judicious removal (over a period of seven months) of the toxic mercury fillings, the Polycythemia vera totally disappeared.

A case in the medical literature, Am J Hematol. 1994 May; 46(1):54-6, revealed a case of "Spontaneous remission of polycythemia vera occurred after 11 years of phlebotomy treatment (blood letting) alone. Sometimes science based medicine does work but takes a little longer.

Case 8. Fifteen Years of Vertigo

A retired school teacher was referred for evaluation and treatment of chronic positional vertigo. The patient stated that he had the vertigo problem for 15 years and was treated by Johns Hopkins and many other prestigious medical centers with science based technology but with no results. Within five minutes of examining the patient, a diagnosis of cytomegalovirus in the inner left ear was made. The source of the virus was a lower left second molar tooth that became toxic following root canal therapy. Two months of treatment using vibrational frequencies and natural nutrients the 15 year duration vertigo totally resolved.

Case 9. Teeth Falling Out of the Jawbone

A 29 year-old woman was referred for examination and treatment of severe generalized bone loss and sudden loss of three molar teeth. Conventional science based medicine could not diagnose the problem. Quantum Medicine technology diagnosed arsenic poisoning, which was confirmed by a hair analysis. The patient's source of arsenic turned out to be the chicken she was eating and vegetables both were severely contaminated with a common pesticide that contained arsenic. The patient was told to modify her diet and include red meat to help rebuild the bone and chelate out the arsenic. Specific natural food-based supplements were prescribed and a bone scan proved scientifically that her bone density improved by 70% in one month with food-based vitamins. It literally took two years of eating a broader type diet assisted with natural nutrients for the patient to regain her full level of health.

Case 10. Idiopathic Tooth Pain

A woman in her early 40's presented with a chief complaint of pain in a tooth for a four year duration. All science based testing proved unsuccessful. Within minutes of using the newer technology, a diagnosis of shingles was made. Three days after treatment with bio-frequencies, the patient's fours years of pain totally resolved.

Case 11. Atypical Facial Pain

Dawn presented with severe facial pain of undetermined origin. Science based medicine could not define the source. Without a diagnosis the patient was subjected to radiosurgery with the gamma knife and when that failed to bring any relief the patient was subjected to major surgery to "alleviate" assumed pressure on the trigeminal nerve (fifth cranial nerve) inside the skull. Both invasive procedures failed to bring any level of pain relief. Comprehensive examination revealed a combination of shingles and herpes simplex I at the apex of the patient's lower right canine tooth, which was treated with root canal therapy. Use of bio-frequencies reduced the pain by 50% in two weeks. After tooth extraction and treatment with ozone, homeopathics, and ionic silver in the surgical extraction site, the severe pain totally resolve.

The key to successful treatment in all cases is to define the core issues. The technologies of advanced Quantum Medicine raises the level of knowledge beyond the capabilities of present day conventional medicine.

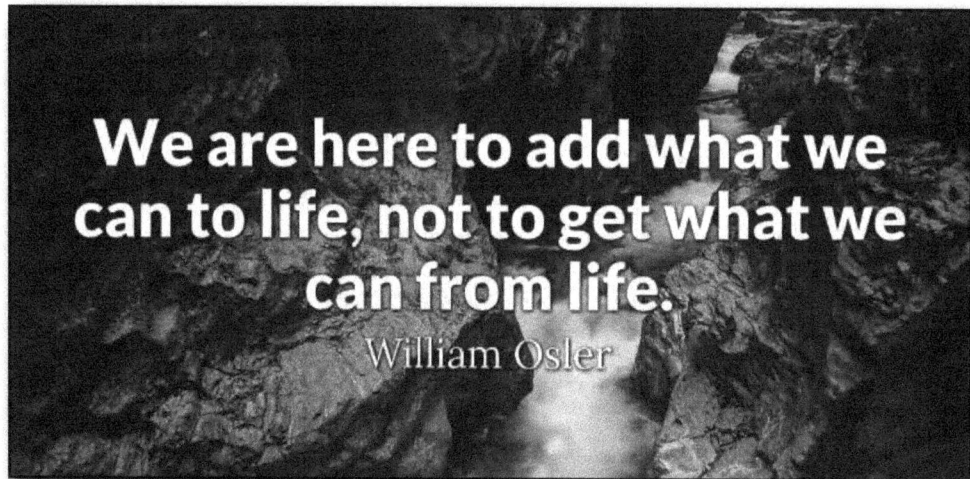

We are here to add what we can to life, not to get what we can from life.
William Osler

1. Yoshiaki Omura, MD and research by Dietrich Klinghardt, M.D., P.h.D. (Autonomic Response Testing), Rheinhold Voll (German medical doctor and acupuncturist), Richard Versendaal, D.C. (Contact Reflex Analysis), Major B. DeJarnette, D.C. (founder of Sacro-Occipital Technique), George Goodheart, D.C. (founder of Applied Kinesiology), Alred C. Fonder, D.D.S. (Originator of the Dental Distress Syndrome),

Basis For Disease

"It's not what you don't know that gets you in trouble, it's what you know for sure that just ain't so."

Mark Twain

Preprogramming Our Subconscious Mind

The noted cellular biologist, Bruce Lipton, Ph.D., in one of his interviews quoted the Jesuit philosophy, "give me a child before the age of seven and I will tell you what kind of adult he or she will be." Unfortunately, like a duck that imprints on its mother, we are all preprogrammed from birth to age seven by what we observe from our family dynamics. This is the reason why many people are resistant to new ideas, change, have negative attitudes and programmed to failure.

Scientific Proof the Germ Theory is Obsolete

Fortunately for society and the goodness of humankind, some of us have chosen to swallow the red pill (Matrix) and break the pattern. Basically, the red pill makes you a rock flipper and puts you on a journey to find the answers to life's many medical mysteries. This has been my journey personally and professionally. The answers are all out there. You just have to become proactive and take the initiative and time to find them.

Most of the disinformation about disease comes from the faulty germ theory that had its inception from Louis Pasteur's research and belief that it was germs that provided the basis for all diseases. In contrast, Pierre Jacques Antoine Béchamp, a French scientist, had an ongoing dispute with Pasteur: he argued vehemently that disease was caused by the pollution of the host's body, milieu, or environment. It has been reported that on his deathbed Pasteur admitted that Béchamp's theory of disease was correct; that it was the polluted body that gave rise to disease and not the germs. Unfortunately, Pasteur's theory became dogma within the medical establishment.

Chapter One

Most secrets of knowledge have been discovered by plain and neglected men rather than by men of popular fame. And this is so with good reason, for the men of popular fame are busy with popular matters.

Roger Bacon (ca. 1220–1292), English philosopher and scientist

In the early 1930s, another genius researcher by the name of Royal Raymond Rife ran experiments which proved that it was the toxic environment that caused healthy bacteria to transmutate into pathogenic forms to causing cancer and disease. He converted a normal healthy bacteria, Bacillus coli, into the BX carcinoma virus 300 times and then reversed the process by changing the medium on which the bacteria and viruses grew. Rife's research proved unequivocally that it was the environment that was the basis for disease. Again, the medical establishment squashed his principles after he successfully treated 16 terminally ill cancer patients and cured every one in 130 days with his frequency generator. The Rife generator was an electronic device that could broadcast specific frequencies that matched the mortal oscillatory frequencies of pathogens. It literally could kill bacteria, viruses, and cancer cells by exploding them without damaging the surrounding healthy cells.

Eleven of the research laboratories that were working to confirm his technology mysteriously burned down within a year. What a coincidence! The tentacles of Big Pharma, the Food and Drug Administration, and the American Medical Association reached out to further suppress the successful cancer study. After the news of the study was published in a San Diego newspaper, the crime syndicate intimidated the three principal doctors who had participated in the cancer research project. When questioned by reporters, all three disavowed knowledge of knowing Dr. Rife, even though they appeared in a photograph with him at the celebration dinner. Dr. E.C. Rosenow, head bacteriologist at the Mayo Clinic, stopped using Dr. Rife's frequency generator and made no future reference to Rife's work. Dr. Arthur Kendall, dean of the Northwestern Medical School, moved to Mexico and lived on his newly acquired 300-acre ranch. Dr. Milbank Johnson, who was the president of the Southern California Medical Society, mysteriously died the night before he was to give a press conference about the cure and recovery of the 16 terminally ill cancer patients. When his body was exhumed six months after his death, they discovered that there was cyanide in his toothpaste. So much for the war on cancer.

In the 1970s, a third researcher, Gaston Naessens, N.D., developed a special light microscope, the somatoscope, which enabled him to discover a new particle in human blood, the somatid. Dr. Naessens discovered that when the medium on which the somatid was growing was altered it transmutated through sixteen different forms to evolve into a pathogenic form. Naessens was also persecuted by the medical establishment for his medical breakthroughs in his successful treatment of cancer, the acquired immunodeficiency syndrome (AIDS), and other immunologically based diseases. In 1985, Naessens was indicted on several counts, the most serious of which carried a potential sentence of life imprisonment. Fortunately, he had many staunch supporters and was brought to trial in Quebec, where he was acquitted and completely exonerated.

In essence, there were three major researchers who confirmed that disease was the result of the pollution of the patient's body and not the direct cause of pathogens. Even with these hardcore scientific findings, present day medical practitioners are still taught that disease is caused by bacteria, viruses, and other mysterious creatures. In fact, Dr. Rife's incredible universal microscope was written up in the Franklin Institute's February 1944 issue of their science journal and yet his name and discoveries have been expunged from all microbiology textbooks.

"Almost no germ is unconditionally dangerous to man; its disease-producing ability depends upon the body's resistance."
Hans Selye, M.D. (International researcher on stress and distress)

For those readers who are still skeptical about the suppression of major breakthroughs in science, I urge you to read the book, *Politics in Healing* by Daniel Haley. Haley gives an in-depth description of five major breakthrough treatments for cancer that were suppressed by the American Medical Association, Big Pharma, and the Food and Drug Administration. The answers to eradicating disease are available but not readily accessible because many practitioners who practice real medicine have been harassed by the establishment, broken financially by bogus lawsuits, and intimidated by fear.

The Fallacious Germ Theory - by JoeDubs

"Germs do not cause disease. The precautions we take to eliminate germs do. These include but are not limited to: antibiotics, disinfectants, food irradiation, hand sanitizers, and vaccines which are designed to protect us from the nefarious germ. We also get sick from our compromised food supply, malnutrition, and inability to recognize what the human body needs.

When we think we "get sick," what is really happening is our bodies are attempting to discard toxic material. "Getting sick" is allowing the body to detoxify itself from toxemia (toxic blood), which is caused by living a toxic life, as well as not absorbing the nutrients our bodies require.

Germs do not cause disease, disease causes germs. Germs are the body's scavengers, the garbage men of your cells. If they are present that means that the conditions where they lie are unfavorable. Change the conditions of the 'terrain', and the germs will morph back into their healthy state.

It is easier for us to put the blame on an outside invader, thereby shifting the responsibility outside of ourselves. But health can only come from within. As Antoine Béchamp said: "Disease is born of us and in us." That same is true for health."

Chapter Two

The Missing Link in Diagnostic Testing

"If I throw a rock out of the window and it goes up instead of down, how many double blind studies do I need to confirm the statistical significance?"

Hans Selye, M.D. (International researcher on stress and distress)

How accurate are laboratory tests? In 1992, a significant study was conducted on 2300 autopsy reports. This study found that the patient's medical histories led to the correct final diagnosis in 76% of the cases, the physical examination did so in 12% of the cases, and the laboratory testing in only 11%.[1] Even the best laboratory tests only reveal reactions to the underlying cause. Just because a mineral like calcium, magnesium, or potassium is outside the normal range, the test does not give you the underlying reason for the abnormality. All the blood testing does is create "analysis paralysis." The key is how to connect the dots to understand what are the real reasons underlying the "disease" process.

After almost fifty years of clinical practice and over 5,000 hours of postgraduate seminars, I have come to the conclusion, that both conventional medicine and many of the alternative disciplines are missing the true diagnostic and treatment links. If a correct diagnosis is not made then the treatment is wrong. Most testing, including blood, kinesiology, energetic, and radiographic, focuses on the patient's normal ranges or physical alterations (broken bones, radiolucencies, tumors, etc.). One must also be aware of the fact that the so-called normal ranges for the blood tests are established from sick people. Why not take the blood ranges from 1,000 healthy Olympic athletes and use them as the basis for establish normal ranges?

1. Peterson MC, Holbrook JH, Hales DV, Smith NL, StakerLV.: Contributions of the history, physical examination, and laboratory investigation in making a medical diagnosis. West J Med. 1992; 156:163-65.

Chapter Two

It wasn't until I entered the realm of energy medicine that I realized that an accurate diagnostic test could be performed to determine the major "splinter(s)" or initiating factor(s) that were corrupting the body's physiology. Clinically I have observed repeatedly that when the "splinters" or initiators are removed, the body reverts back to "factory default." It is just like pushing the reset button on your electronic device. The body wants to go back to normal, but the initiators are preventing it. The closer one gets to the truth, the more simplistic the solution.

"If you don't read the newspaper, you are uninformed. If you do read the newspaper, you are misinformed." *Mark Twain*

Unfortunately this quotation holds true for many medical journals today.

Eleven Year-Old's Severe Eczema Resolved with Energy Medicine Diagnostics and Nutritional Protocol

Debunking the Latest Medical Mantra for Plaque Psoriasis, Eczema and Rashes

After practicing 50 years, I have come to realize that the medical industry has been practicing "fake medicine." Treating symptoms with drugs to control symptoms is not healing but quackery. In addition, one must also pay close attention to the "safety considerations" related to the drug du jour. In most cases, taking the "cure" exposes you to potentially deadly consequences. Just read the warning accompanying Humira, the latest drug in a mass television campaign focusing on plaque psoriasis.

Safety Considerations

Serious infections have happened in people taking HUMIRA. These serious infections include tuberculosis (TB) and infections caused by viruses, fungi, or bacteria that have spread throughout the body. Some people have died from these infections. HUMIRA may increase the chance of getting lymphoma, including a rare kind, or other cancers. HUMIRA can cause serious side effects including hepatitis B infection in carriers of the virus, allergic reactions, nervous system problems, blood problems, heart failure, certain immune reactions including a lupus-like syndrome, liver problems, and new or worsening psoriasis.

Cancer—for children and adults taking tumor necrosis factor (TNF) blockers, including HUMIRA, the chance of getting lymphoma or other cancers may increase. There have been cases of unusual cancers in children, teenagers, and young adults using TNF blockers. Some people have developed a rare type of cancer called hepatosplenic T-cell lymphoma. This type of cancer often results in death. If using TNF blockers including HUMIRA, your chance of getting two types of skin cancer (basal cell and squamous cell) may increase. These types are generally not life-threatening if treated; tell your doctor if you have a bump or open sore that doesn't heal.

Real healing must focus on uncovering the underlying cause. When the second largest excretory gland of the body, the skin, exhibits symptoms (rashes, acne, plaque psoriasis, blisters, etc.), one must look at the potential causes: issues with the liver, thyroid, gallbladder, intestines, kidneys, lungs, and other organs plus chemicals (pesticides, PCBs, dioxin, fluoride, etc.), heavy metals (mercury, cadmium, aluminum, lead, arsenic, etc.), drugs and vaccines that may become trapped within the skin. A perfect example is the case of an eleven year-old Amish boy who was referred to my office for evaluation and treatment of severe eczema. The lesions were present for over a year and many medical specialists were consulted. Unfortunately the topical steroids, antibiotics and other type medicaments had no lasting effect. Because the list of potential causative items mentioned are not in the vocabulary of traditional medicine they didn't even entertain the idea to even look for these items.

Reversing Severe Eczema

Using energetic medicine and Direct Resonance Testing techniques the following factors were found within the eczema: herpes zoster, herpes simplex I, and cytomegalovirus. In addition, the patient had a low thyroid function, which lowered his immune system preventing resolution of the pathogens. A nutritional program was set up which addressed detoxing his liver, opening up his avenues of excretion, reducing heavy metals, and neutralizing the vaccines with homeopathic nosodes and herbs known to be affective agains viruses. The comprehensive approach totally resolved the severe eczema in three months. Interestingly, there were no known side effects of the remedies that could cause TB, bacterial, viral or fungal infections or the potential of causing cancer. Why would anyone subject themselves to these dangers when a safer, more effective approach is available?

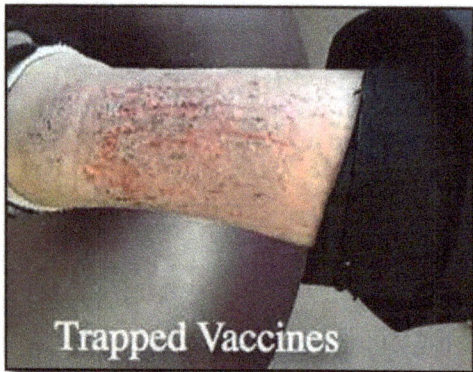

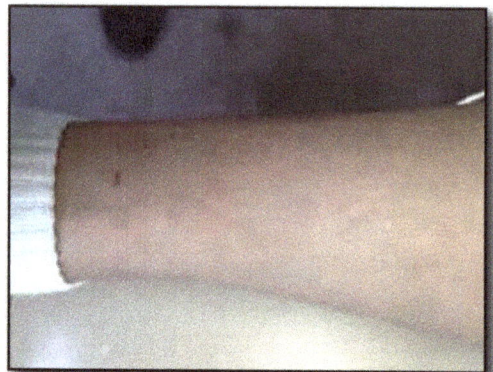

Before and after images. 3 months Tx; Nutritional Support vitamins, herbs and homeopathics. Must use food-based remedies for maximum results

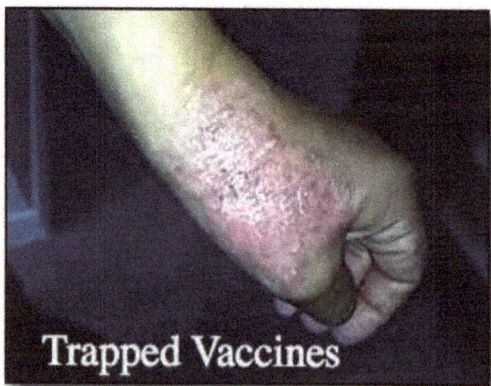

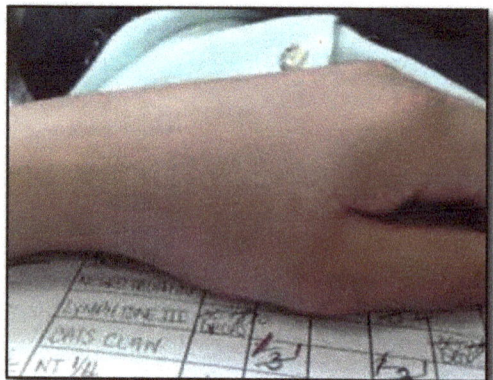

As was brought home to us in spades through the recent election cycle, virtually all traditional media spews out "fake news" about politics and economics with agendas geared to manipulating public opinion. Why would we think their agendas are any less-fake when it comes to reporting on health and medical issues? No different than the political establishment, the medical industry, through the media, feeds us "fake" or disinformation regarding issues ranging from the "war" on cancer, vaccine safety (the FDA recently admitted they have not submitted a safety report in over thirty years, and the deaths attributed to adverse reactions are much higher than they reported), Vioxx efficacy, how effective statins are for cholesterol and the drug du jour are for plaque psoriasis, eczema, and other common symptoms. Hopefully, the public at large is awakening to the tragedies fostered by "fake news."

Based on quantum physics, everything in the universe has an energetic signature. Just as there are no two finger-prints that are exactly alike, so too there are no energetic duplications of physical signature identities. Utilizing the quantum testing (Bi-digital "O" ring test) concepts developed by Yoshiaki Omura, M.D., one can use a test vial with a known imprinted frequency of a specific substance to diagnostically determine if that substance (chemical, vaccine, virus, bacteria, pesticide, heavy metal, etc.) is present in a particular part of the body. What an ingenious concept. It's quick, accurate, instantaneous, noninvasive, less costly to the patient, and best of all it identifies the initiating factor(s). In essence, a physiologic diagnosis is made. In comparison an oncologist makes a histologic diagnosis, which describes to the "nth" degree of detail the size of the tumor, the arrangement of the cells, whether the stroma is mixoid, or the mucosa ulcerated, and so on, but nowhere in the report does it even mention there are heavy metals, pesticides, viruses, or chemicals that represent the real underlying diagnostic value. The following case studies provide perfect examples of the validity of a physiologic diagnosis as opposed to a histologic diagnosis.

Lung Cancer

Carol K. was referred to my office because she had lung cancer in her right lung. The oncologic surgeon removed the tip of her right lung where the cancer was located. Six months later, the cancer reappeared in the upper portion of her left lung. One has to realize that cutting out the cancer is like painting over rust. The real cause is not being addressed. The patient rejected the recommended second surgery and chemotherapy treatments. On her second visit, I requested the patient to bring in her histologic slides of the cancer. Energetic testing of the actual tissue revealed the presence of a pesticide, cytomegalovirus, and mercury. A nutritional program was initiated and specific supplements were prescribed to detoxify the liver and the three splinters in the cancerous tissue, re-establish intestinal balance, and regenerate the cells back to "factory default." In six months the cancer in the left lung had totally disappeared, as stated in the hospital's own records. The concept is simple and hidden in plain view. Remove the "splinter(s)" and allow the tissues to heal.

Canine Lip Cancer

One of my patients brought her labradoodle in for diagnosis and treatment of lip cancer. The dog had been surgically treated by Cornell Veterinary Hospital. Twice the oncologic veterinarian surgically removed the cancer and twice the cancer returned. I proceeded to evaluate the dog using test kits with known frequencies of specific initiators (e.g. viruses, heavy metals, chemicals, pesticides). A definitive diagnosis was made. The area of the cancer contained a specific virus, heavy metal, and a pesticide. The dog was placed on a prescribed supplement program to remove the offending initiators and simultaneously detox him. In six weeks on the program, the dog's lip cancer "fell" off.

Stage Four Throat Cancer

When Roland told his endocrinologist he was going to go alternative to treat his stage four throat cancer, the physician told him alternative treatment was a farce and that he would be wasting his time and money. When Roland was examined, he had three root canal teeth that radiographically looked pristine. However, when tested energetically the three teeth had specific pathogens that were also present in the exact area of the cancer. Interestingly, the patient asked how he would chew of he lost the three teeth. I replied if you die it won't make a difference. Roland got the message, and agreed to have the three teeth removed. Immediately following extractions, the surgical site was meticulously curetted to remove any periodontal ligaments and debris, soft bone was removed, and the area was irrigated with ozone, colloidal silver, and Sanum homeopathic remedies. The sockets were also packed with Gelfoam (resorbable sponge) that was saturated with homeopathic remedies. The patient was also placed on a raw food diet, supplements, and told to use Rife frequencies to kill the pathogens. He was also undergoing insulin potentiation treatment (IPT) at the time. IPT therapy works by lowering the blood sugar levels with intravenous insulin to starve the cancer cells; this technique enables administration of a chemotherapeutic agent at one-tenth the normal dose. The cancer cells ingest the chemotherapy agent along with an administered sugar, and effectively kills the cancer cells. In three weeks, after removing the "splinters," the patient's stage four throat cancer totally disappeared. When Roland confronted his endocrinologist about speaking to his other cancer patients to apprise them of alternative therapies, the doctor would not respond. So much for the "Hippocratic Oath."

The concept of defining and removing the underlying "splinter(s)" has also been successfully applied to many other medical maladies (e.g., Hashimoto's disease, Raynaud's disease, hormonal migraines, asthma, allergies, vertigo, eczema, and atypical facial pain). The problem with the paradigm is that it is too simple. In addition to removing the primary causative factors, the three pillars of health must also be addressed. Without changing the terrain, the disease process will continue with dire consequences.

High Blood Pressure Resolved With Systemic Enzymes

When there is an oversupply of sodium in the extracellular fluids, the kidneys will initially expel the excess sodium. If the kidneys fail to expel the sodium from the blood, the peripheral vascular system will constrict and the resistance to blood flow will increase, the result is high blood pressure.

In order to control this, the medical profession introduced diuretics to treat high blood pressure. In diuretics, more fluid is expelled from the body together with sodium chloride. This is effective in the early stage of high blood pressure. However, the kidneys are also required to expel potassium, hence the deficiency in potassium. As a remedy, doctors should prescribe potassium supplements and drinking of plenty of water as replenishments.

Another major factor in high blood pressure is inflammation. Processed foods especially junk food in particular and even many good restaurants have one thing in common, they use adulterated oils for cooking. Adulterated seed oils such as sunflower, safflower, corn, grapeseed, soy, canola and vegetable oils (usually soy) are all high in omega-6 (linoleic acid). When these adulterated oils enter the body and become impregnated into the cell membranes of the intima (inner blood vessel lining) they cause inflammation which narrow the lumen of the blood vessel and raises blood pressure.

The key point is that physicians are not getting to the root cause of the high blood pressure issue but only treating the symptom. One major component that is not even considered is the deposition of fibrin in the micro capillaries through out the body. When these small blood vessels clog up, the heart has to pump harder to get the blood into the tissues thus elevating the blood pressure. A more logical approach would be to dissolve the fibrin out of the capillaries. This can easily be accomplished using serrapeptase, an enzyme produced by the silk worm.

Two cases in point. One patient had consistently high blood pressure (180/92). The patient was prescribed all the prescription drugs (diuretics and even calcium channel blockers) in an attempt to control his blood pressure but nothing worked. The patient even tried numerous natural remedies but they did not work either. After just eight weeks on the systemic enzyme, serrapeptase, his blood pressure normalized.

The other patient had spiking of his blood pressure (145/93 - 130/80) during the day. Again all attempts to normalize his pressure failed. The patient was diagnosed with parasites in his small intestines. Within ninety days after taking a tablespoon of food grade diatomaceous earth daily in twelve ounces of water, his blood pressure normalized with no spiking (112/76).

Like any medical condition, the practitioner ultimately must get to the underlying cause. Unfortunately, our medical system focuses primarily on symptomatic treatment and the patient is left with a false sense of security that his medical condition is under control.

The Three Pillars to Achieve Ultimate Health

Establishing health involves a three-prong approach: detoxification, rebalancing the intestinal flora, and regeneration.

When treating patients, a comprehensive biological approach is the key to achieving a successful outcome. Detoxification is essential for cleaning the primary filter, the liver, as well as removing other diagnosed toxins. When the milieu or body's environment becomes polluted, healthy microbes transmutate into pathologic forms. This metamorphosis was well documented by Dr. Royal Raymond Rife back in the 1930s and again in the 1970s by Dr. Gaston Naessens.

Chapter Two

Even Louis Pasteur admitted on his deathbed that Antoine Béchamp's concept of a polluted terrain as being the cause of disease was correct.

The toxic initiators of the disease process are many. Heavy metals, pesticides, chemicals, pathogens, acid pH, vaccines and their adjuvants, psychological distress, genetically modified foods, chemtrails, chlorinated and fluoridated water, electromagnetic frequencies, gluten, foods high in phytoestrogen (soy, flax oil, etc.), high fructose corn syrup, dental infections (root canals, cavitations, galvanic currents, toxic dental materials, tooth decay), and pharmaceuticals are just a few toxins that practitioners should make a conscious effort to diagnose and reduce. These toxic initiators disrupt the normal physiology of the cells, tissues, organs, and alter the DNA. The ultimate result is systemic inflammation, which in turn causes fibrosis. It is the fibrosis that reduces the micro-circulation and normal cell function. The end result is degeneration, disease, and death.

Removing the initiators enables the liver to more efficiently filter the blood, thereby providing cells with an abundance of oxygen, nutrients, and waste removal, all required to maintain homeostasis. In addition, the immune system can more effectively remove cancer cells, pathogens, and other foreign materials.

Psychological distress plus the presence of initiators produce a common symptom, systemic inflammation, particularly in the intestines, which provide 60 to 80 percent of the body's immune system. Swelling of the intestinal mucosa, which includes Peyer's patches, reduces the immune system by one-third to one half of its effectiveness. Without removing the initiators and inflammation, one can never resolve the physiologic dysfunction.

The first objective is to remove the causative factor(s) and reduce the distress as much as possible. Once the intestinal inflammation subsides, the healthy flora can be reintroduced by means of pre-and probiotics. A diet high in fiber, devoid of dairy, sugar, and wheat (gluten) will dramatically reduce the slugging of the lymphatic or drainage system of the body. A cleaner intestine insures better nutrient absorption and healthier cells. Once the burden of toxins is reduced and the intestinal mucosa is restored, it is time to regenerate the cells, tissues and organs. By supplying protomorphogens, genetic blue-prints provided by desiccated bovine tissue, the body can start repairing the damage. Homeopathic sarcodes (remedies that stimulate normal function), food-based nutrients, and raw foods provide the building blocks for repair. Restoring the three pillar's of health is your insurance policy for maintaining a quality of life. The closer one gets to the truth, the more simplistic the solution. A biological approach to healing meets the physiologic needs of the body and has a formative tract record to support its principles.

Inflammation - The Underlying Cause for All Diseases

Inflammation is the common denominator of all diseases! The National Council on Aging reports that a shocking 80 percent of people 65 and over suffer from at least one condition (arthritis, cancer, diabetes, and Crohn's)

Inflammation is the body's attempt at self-protection; its aim is to remove harmful stimuli, including damaged cells, irritants, and pathogens - and begin the healing process. This response to tissue injury functions to limit the damaged area and remove (or prevent the spread of) a pathogenic agent.

Thomas Sydenham, a Cambridge University scholar, gave his opinion about the inflammatory process: " A disease is the effort of nature to restore the health of the patient by elimination of morbific matter." In essence, what Sydenham was saying was that inflammation was not a pathological entity attempting to destroy life, but as a mechanism of repair in an effort to sustain life.

An example of this healing process is fever. Most authorities and laypersons believe that body temperatures below 106^0 F are harmless and those above 108^0 F are potentially harmful. A study conducted by Dr. Barton D. Schmitt, University of Colorado pediatrician suggested that doctors reeducate parents about fever. He established that misguided parents are overly concerned about fever in children to the point they have a fever phobia and as a result, treat fevers overaggressively. Dr. Schmitt stated that fever rarely produces serious complications (Am J Disease Child, 1980). Medical records show that more than one person has sustained fever as high as 114.8^0 F without suffering the greatly feared brain damage.

Warning:

A double-blind study conducted by Dr. O.P.J. Falk found that flu patients given aspirin were disabled twice as long and had 3.5 times more complications as those who were given sugar pills. Aspirin will make you worse by increasing the cell membrane permeability enabling the virus to spread more easily.

Inflammation is the body's immune response to a tissue injury or an invasion by foreign agents, such as viruses, bacteria, other microorganisms, chemicals, pesticides, heavy metals, vaccines and toxins (mercaptans, hydrogen sulfide, and thioethers) from root canal teeth. It is a protective mechanism that our body uses to remove the pathological agent and initiate tissue repair. However, this is a temporary mechanism and inflammation can turn into pathology if it becomes excessive and chronic. Long lasting inflammation can trigger cascades of various biological signal responses which initiate abnormal cellular activities in neighboring tissues and cells leading to damage of healthy cells and tissue.

Inflammation can occur suddenly as an acute reaction, such as a response to injury. The symptoms are heat, redness, swelling, and pain in the affected area. Inflammation can also persist for a long time in relation to lasting infection, ulceration, irritation or autoimmune disease, and can become a chronic process. Such inflammation is often the foundation for many chronic degenerative diseases that take years to develop. Chronic inflammation in the joints leads to arthritis, in the membranes around the heart to pericarditis, and in the stomach it causes gastritis. Inflammation accompanies chronic pain, asthma, multiple sclerosis, atherosclerosis, cancer, and many other diseases.

Causes of Inflammation:
1. Wounds
2. Heavy metals (mercury, arsenic, cadmium, aluminum, nickel, lead)
3. Chemicals (dioxins, PCBs, chlorine, fluoride, bromine)
4. Pathogens: viruses, bacteria, mold, fungi
5. Vaccinations: specially the adjuvants (formaldehyde, Al, Hg, polysorbitol 80, fetal tissue, retrovirus contamination).
6. Eating rancid or oxidized omega-6 oils (corn, soy, safflower, sunflower, canola)
7. Eating refined sugar encourages inflammation and cancer growth.

8. Mercury toxicity from dental amalgams, contaminated fish, and coal burning power plants.

9. Herbicides especially glyphosate (Round-Up) are endocrine disrupters (increase estrogen)

10. Hypothyroidism

11. Vitamin and minerals deficiencies: B-complex, vitamin A, vitamin C, Vitamin E, and essential fatty acids

12. High Fructose corn syrup

13. Smoking

14. Periodontal disease (gum disease)

15. Stress

16. Sedentary life style

17. Toxic root canal teeth (mercaptans, hydrogen sulfide, thioethers)

18. EMFs: over use of cell phones with headsets

19. Chronic infections

20. Eating too much processed foods (grains, pastries, pastas)

21. Parasites: Giardia, amoeba, pin worms, cryptosporidium

22. Systemic candida

23. Dehydration: fluid not getting inside the cells

24. Fluoride: Fluoride depresses thyroid activity; impaired antioxidant defense systems

25. Poor digestion

26. Abnormal insulin levels: diabetes

27. Food allergies

28. Body Ph too acidic: diet high in refined foods

30. Genetically modified foods (soy, wheat, corn)

31. Galvanic currents from dissimilar metals: surgical stainless steel pins, titanium implants and gold crowns. All are connected via the body fluids which creates a battery effect

32. Sympathetic dominance (flight or fight reaction): causes the intercellular fluids to gel trapping toxins and waste products

33. Hormone imbalance specially elevated estrogen levels: bisphenol A (synthetic estrogen) from soft plastic containers, plastic liners in canned foods

34. Nutritional deficiencies Vitamin C (scurvy); Vitamin A and E (allergies); Vitamin E (heart inflammation due to poor quality of the food)

35. Dysbiosis of the intestinal flora: gluten-laden foods and Round-Up (glyphosate) – which can cause "leaky gut" syndrome, an increased permeability of the intestinal lining, that cause all kinds of health issues like, depression, anxiety, thyroid disorders – to name just a few.

The Difference Between Chronic and Acute Inflammation

If you have an injury or infection, inflammation is necessary to help protect and heal your body. Through a series of biochemical reactions, white blood cells and other chemicals are sent to the injured area to fight off foreign bodies.

You've certainly experienced this type of beneficial acute inflammation if you've had a cut or infection, and the symptoms typically include:
redness, warmth, pain, swelling, and loss of movement and function.

When inflammation becomes chronic, there are often no symptoms until a loss of function occurs. This is because chronic inflammation is low-grade and systemic, often silently damaging your tissues. This process can go on for years without you noticing, until a disease such as heart disease, cancer, Alzheimer's or autoimmune disease like multiple sclerosis, ulcerative colitis, or rheumatoid arthritis develops.
`

What Causes Chronic Inflammation?

Chronic inflammation can be the result of a malfunctioning, over-reactive immune system, or it may be due to an underlying problem that your body is attempting to fight off. Many of these "problems" are actually due to an unhealthy lifestyle.

Chronic inflammation promotes the production of free radicals, which play a role in causing cancer, diabetes, and cardiovascular disease.

Clinical biomarkers of inflammation are used to study the effect of dietary constituents on inflammation. C-reactive protein (CRP), which is an acute phase reactant protein, is a common clinical biomarker of cardiac-related inflammation and also a general marker of inflammation. Other common clinical indicators of inflammation are a high erythrocyte sedimentation rate (ESR), a high white blood cell count, and a low albumin level. However, these tests are nonspecific, meaning an abnormal result might result from a condition unrelated to inflammation.

Conventional Medicine: Patients suffering from inflammatory disorders often take painkillers in order to alleviate the pain. While these drugs can decrease the suffering from pain, they do not eliminate the cause of the inflammation. Treatments that target inflammation involve the use of synthetic steroids and a family of "non-steroidal anti-inflammatory drugs" (NSAIDS) both of which have many undesirable side effects. NSAIDS are widely used especially for a variety of muscle and joint problems. These drugs inhibit the enzymes that are necessary for the formation of prostaglandins. Prostaglandins are one of a number of hormone-like substances that participate in a wide range of body functions such as the contraction and relaxation of smooth muscle, the dilation and constriction of blood vessels, control of blood pressure, and modulation of inflammation. Prostaglandins are derived from a chemical called arachidonic acid (present in chicken soup).

While they may help in relieving symptoms they also have negative health effects. The most serious and life threatening side effect of NSAIDS are gastrointestinal complications, such as bleeding. Never use an over-the-counter NSAID for more than 10 days without checking with your doctor. Over-the-counter NSAIDs are effective pain relievers, but they are intended for short-term use.

A new class of drugs called COX2 inhibitors (such as VIOXX) was not associated with this problem; however, VIOXX was taken off the market because it increased the risk of death from heart attacks.

Cellular medicine research: Various scientific studies have shown that proper nutrition helps in controlling inflammation and that some micronutrient deficiencies (i.e., vitamin A) can aggravate existing inflammatory responses.

Studies have found that **diets high in saturated fat and trans fat** are pro-inflammatory in nature. In contrast, some studies have found that adherence to a Mediterranean-style diet — a diet high in monounsaturated fats — may help reduce inflammation. A Mediterranean diet emphasizes olive oil, fruit and vegetables, nuts, beans, fish, whole grains, and moderate consumption of alcohol. Several of these foods are important sources of essential fatty acids that are involved in the inflammatory process. Higher intake of the omega-3 fatty acids can be obtained from:

- Cold water high-fat fish, especially wild Alaskan salmon, sardines, anchovies, mackerel, shad, herring, and trout
- Flaxseed oil (which has the highest linolenic content of any food), flaxseeds, flaxseed meal, hempseed oil, hemp seeds, walnuts, pumpkin seeds, Brazil nuts, and sesame seeds
- Avocados
- Certain dark green leafy vegetables, including kale, spinach, purslane, mustard greens, and collards

The omega-3 fatty acids have been generally associated with decreased biomarkers of inflammation.

Rich dietary sources of omega-6 oils include:

- Safflower, sunflower, sesame oil, and walnuts and their oil
- Grapeseed oil
- Pumpkin seeds

- Pignolia (pine) nuts and pistachios
- Borage oil, evening primrose oil, black currant seed oil

All seeds must be organic, raw and the oils must be organic and cold pressed to be biologically active.

On average, the body's tissues have an 11 to 1 ratio of omega-6 to omega-3 fatty acids. The omega-6s line the entire gastrointestinal tract and inner lining of the blood vessels. It is the omega-6 oil that acts as a magnet in the cell membranes to pull in the oxygen. This is one of the most important factors in maintaining cellular health.

Micronutrients

Several micronutrients are related to diseases that have inflammatory components, e.g., cardiovascular disease, type 2 diabetes, inflammatory bowel disease, chronic obstructive pulmonary disease (COPD), and rheumatoid arthritis.

Vitamin A (beef lipid source not fish oil)

Dr. Eli Seifter, Ph.D, associate professor of Biochemistry, Albert Einstein College of Medicine, wrote that vitamin A increases the immune response and shortens the duration of the illness. *All fish oils go rancid at room temperature! They also suppress the energy production in the heart mitochondria, which can cause a heart attack.*

Magnesium

A U.S. national survey, found that 75% of American adults consumed less than the RDA of magnesium and were 1.48 to 1.75 times more likely to have an elevated C-reactive protein level (indicative of systemic inflammation) compared to those who consumed at least the RDA recommendation: 310 - 420mg. This survey found that 68% of the sample consumed less than the RDA of magnesium. Magnesium is active in over 73% of the enzymatic reactions; it's present in green leafy vegetables.

Vitamin B6

Low vitamin B6 status was associated with higher C-reactive protein levels; a low circulating level of vitamin B6 is a risk factor for cardiovascular disease. It helps the body make the hormones serotonin (which regulates mood) and norepinephrine (which helps your heart beat strongly and your body cope with stress). The body needs all the B vitamins and not just fractionated isolated ones.

Vitamin C

Adequate dietary intake of the food based antioxidant vitamin C, is also important because free radicals have pro-inflammatory effects. Higher vitamin C levels were also associated with lower C-reactive protein levels. Vitamin C is anti-inflammatory, anti-viral, anti-bacterial, anti-fungal and may help protect against diseases with inflammatory components such as coronary heart disease and gout.

Vitamin D$_3$

Several human studies associated vitamin D$_3$ deficiency or impaired vitamin D$_3$ status with various inflammatory diseases, such as Crohn's disease and other inflammatory bowel diseases. Vitamin D$_3$ status may also be linked to cardiovascular disease and certain cancers. Vitamin D$_3$ levels for a healthy adult should range from 50 ng/mL - 70 ng/mL. Cancer patients require a higher range, 70 ng/mL to 100 ng/mL, to be effective in supporting the immune system.

Osteoporosis: hypothyroidism and vitamin D$_3$ insufficiency can be important etiological factors in older adults. Osteoporosis affects one-third of women aged 60-70 years and two-thirds of women aged 80 years and above. A multinational (18 different countries with latitudes ranging from 64 degrees north to 38 degrees south) survey of more than 2,600 postmenopausal women with osteoporosis revealed that 64% of subjects had 25-hydroxy vitamin D$_3$ levels lower than 30 ng/

mL in a recent case-control study that included 111 hip fracture patients and 73 controls (median age, 83 years) found low serum levels of both 25-hydroxy vitamin D_3 and vitamin K were associated with an increased risk of hip fracture. Without sufficient vitamin D_3 from sun exposure or dietary intake, intestinal calcium absorption can be significantly reduced.

Cancer

A recent systematic review and meta-analysis of 16 prospective studies, including 137,567 subjects, reported an 11% reduction in total cancer incidence and a 17% reduction in cancer mortality with each 20 ng/mL increase in circulating 25-hydroxy vitamin D_3 levels. Numerous experimental studies have demonstrated that biologically active forms of vitamin D_3 can control cell fate by inhibiting proliferation and/or inducing cell differentiation or death (apoptosis) of a number of cancerous cell types. Vitamin D_3 levels for a healthy adult: 50 - 70 ng/mL; for cancer patients 70 -100 ng/mL.

Vitamin E

Vitamin E has effects on inflammatory processes due to the antioxidant functions of α-tocopherol. α-Tocopherol exerts anti-inflammatory effects through a number of different mechanisms, for example, by decreasing levels of C-reactive protein and pro-inflammatory cytokines. University studies have also documented the positive effect of delta-tocopherol against cancer cells. To be effective, delta-tocopherols must be taken several hours away from any other vitamin E formula.

Carotenoids

Carotenoids, the yellow, orange, and red pigments synthesized by plants, have a number of different biological activities. Carotenoid β-carotene displayed anti-inflammatory activity by inhibiting pro-inflammatory gene expression. The carotenoids, lycopene and astaxanthin, have also been shown to exhibit anti-inflammatory activities in cell cultures and animal models. Sources of lycopene include tomatoes, red grapefruit, red watermelon, and guava, while the main dietary sources of astaxanthin include salmon, shrimp, and other seafood.

Flavonoids

Another class of phytochemicals with anti-inflammatory effects includes the flavonoids. Various flavonoids, such as quercetin, kaempferol, and genistein, possess anti-inflammatory properties.

Other dietary phytochemicals

Resveratrol is a polyphenolic compound naturally found in peanuts, grapes, red wine, and some berries.

Two randomized, placebo-controlled trials reported that one-year consumption of a grape supplement containing 8 mg/day of resveratrol improved inflammatory and atherogenic status in subjects at risk for cardiovascular disease, as well as in patients with established coronary heart disease.

Other phytochemicals, namely curcumin, ginger and garlic-derived compounds, have been shown to exhibit anti-inflammatory properties.

α-Lipoic acid is a naturally occurring compound that is synthesized in small amounts by the body. It is also obtained in the diet from tomatoes, green leafy vegetables, cruciferous vegetables, and other sources. Endogenous α-lipoic acid functions as a cofactor for mitochondrial enzymes important in the generation of energy. When provided as a dietary supplement, however, α-lipoic acid may display a number of other biological activities, including antioxidant and anti-inflammatory functions. Results from studies in cell cultures and animal models have shown the compound has anti-inflammatory properties, but human data are extremely limited. A small placebo-controlled trial in patients with metabolic syndrome found that supplementation with α-lipoic acid (300 mg/day) for four weeks resulted in a 15% decline in plasma levels of interleukin-6, an inflammatory marker of atherosclerosis.

Natural Ways to Reduce Inflammation

- Detox: natural herbal teas: Essiac (turkey rhubarb, slippery elm, burdock, and sheep sorrel); herbs: turmeric, garlic, milk thistle, cilantro; vitamins: glutathione, SOD, vitamins C, A, and E.
- Eat organic foods: avocado, almonds, carrots, beets, pineapple, radishes.
- Eat more dark green leafy vegetables: Kale, collard greens, BokChoy, celery, dandelion greens
- Drink water (coffee, tea, sodas do NOT count as liquids); specially structured water and/ or hydrogen water.

Lifestyle Factors

Animal and human studies have found that various forms of physical activity decrease both acute and chronic inflammation, as measured by reductions in C-reactive protein and certain pro-inflammatory cytokines. Moreover, regular physical activity is important in reducing one's risk for obesity and chronic diseases associated with inflammation. However, *excessive exercise can increase systemic inflammation.* For example, overtraining syndrome in athletes is associated with systemic inflammation and suppressed immune function. Several studies have shown that moderate alcohol consumption decreases risk of cardiovascular disease, as well as all-causes of mortality. Further, smoking cessation has been reported to decrease C-reactive protein and other biomarkers of inflammation.

The reader should walk away with the understanding that reducing inflammation is good, however, the source of the inflammation must also be removed to effect true healing.

"The good physician treats the disease; the great physician treats the patient who has the disease."

Sir William Osler

Chapter Four - Cranial Complex

Comprehensive Testing System - The Cranial Complex

The noted psychologist, Edward de Bono, stated that to solve complex problems one must engage in lateral thinking. There are no magic bullets. In order to solve complex problems, one must integrate the various disciplines to decipher the underlying cause(s).

Forty-eight years into clinical practice and thirty-five years of research studying osteopathic, chiropractic, dental, medical, physical therapy, and nutritional concepts, the light bulb finally went on. Practitioners must approach patients' chief complaints by evaluating them in five major areas: Cranial Complex, Dental Complex, Pelvic Complex, Physiological Complex, and Psychological Complex. A patient's symptoms can originate in any one or a combination of the above categories.

The cranium presents a magnificent architectural masterpiece of design features that enable human kind to survive the rigors of life. The sutures between the individual cranial bones act as expansion-contraction joints to allow the skull to accommodate changes in barometric pressure and withstand traumas. When the sutures are locked up, patient complaints of severe headaches are a great predictor of days before a storm front arrives. When the barometric pressure drops prior to a storm, and if the skull bones are restricted in their normal motion, pain is elicited from the compression within the sutures. The same response occurs when flying. If the persons' skull bones are restricted, he or she will experience nausea when the plane is taking off and landing. The cranium elicits parasympathetic stimulation via the vagus nerve, which causes bile and digestive juices to flow. On an empty stomach or even when the stomach is full, excess fluids and vagal stimulation will cause nausea.

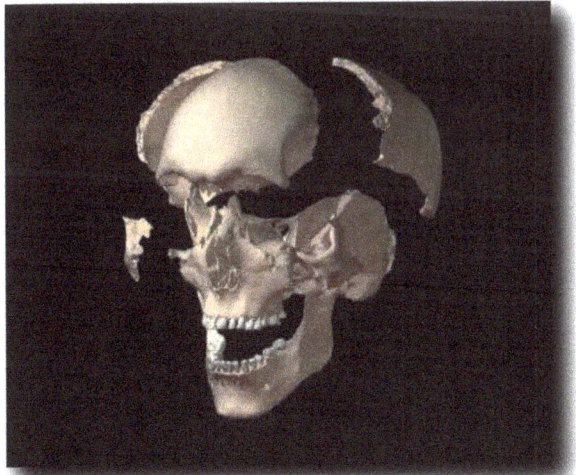

Chapter Four - Cranial Complex

In addition, trauma to the skull is dissipated by both the ability of the sutures to absorb the forces encountered and by the buttresses provided by the lateral arches (zygomatic arches or cheek bones) of the cranium. Even the teeth have a fail safe mechanism against trauma. They are attached to their sockets by means of periodontal ligaments which act as shock absorbers. Furthermore, the cerebrospinal fluid that surrounds the brain acts like a cushion during impact.

Symptoms that may relate to cranial distortions may be caused by head trauma, orthodontic braces, Invisalign, malocclusion, whiplash, tooth extraction, wisdom teeth removal, root canal treatment, mouth trauma, oral infections, mercury fillings, tooth implants, dental bridgework, partial dentures, full dentures, loss of vertical height of the teeth (due to wear or faulty restoration), occlusal equilibration (grinding the teeth to adjust the bite), and resin fillings (white material). The aforementioned procedures or events are those that should motivate the physician to consider evaluating the cranium, since they may relate to the patient's chief complaints:

- Headaches (tension, migraines, cluster, ophthalmic)
- Dizziness
- Disequilibrium or balance problems
- Visual distortions
- Post-concussion symptoms
- Insomnia
- Fatigue
- Mental fog
- Anxiety, depression, and panic attacks
- Poor memory
- Atypical facial pain
- Seizures
- Alzheimer's disease

- Parkinson's disease
- ALS (amyotrophic lateral sclerosis)
- MS (multiple sclerosis)
- Agitation
- Bipolar disorder
- Attention Deficit Disorder, attention deficit/hyperactivity disorder
- Autistic spectrum
- Allergies
- Cervical/neck pain
- Low back pain
- Swollen lymph nodes
- Nausea

Another area of concern is contamination of the brain from vaccines and their adjuvants, and infections in the brain such as Lyme's disease or from cytomegalovirus, herbicides (especially glyphosate [Monsanto's Round-Up)], heavy metals, chemicals; even prescription medications can get trapped within the brain tissue. I recently had a case in which the patient was diagnosed with Alzheimer's disease. When he was energetically tested, glyphosate, mercury, and Lyme infection showed up in his left frontal cortex area. Appropriate treatment with specific nutrients to remove the "splinters" brought dramatic results. The patient became much more alert; he was able to speak more clearly; able to follow instructions more easily, and he was more in the present and without having that glazed look in his eyes.

Child's Seizures Following Four-Month Schedule of Vaccines
How Safe is Your Child's Vaccine?

An eight-month-old male infant was referred to me for evaluation of seizures. The child developed seizures and became noninteractive shortly after his four-month schedule of vaccines. From birth to six months the recommended vaccine schedule includes hepatitis B, rotavirus, diphtheria, pertussis, tetanus, and pneumococcal vaccine. The pediatrician referred the child to a major children's hospital where they put him on steroids to treat the seizures. He became wired and irritable. Since he was not showing any improvement, the parents decided to take a more natural approach.

The initial evaluation revealed a viral meningococcal infection in the left side of the brain along with thimerosal (ethyl mercury), glyphosate (herbicide Round-Up) cadmium, aluminum, and lead. A nutritional program was prescribed and tested for compatibility. Within six weeks the child's seizures resolved and he became the loving interactive child he had been prior to the vaccines. The two critical points are: 1) vaccines are dangerous, especially with all the toxic additives, and 2) conventional treatment for this condition is obsolete and has potentially dangerous side effects.

UPDATE
Why Corporate Medicine is a Poor Investment
The little toddler is now 10.5 months old. In June 2018, he spent 5 days in Children's Hospital of Philadelphia (CHOPS), where they ran an Epilepsy Panel as well as numerous other tests. You can be sure the tab for his visit was well over $50,000. The result of his evaluation was that he was placed on a steroid to reduce the inflammation in his brain. Unfortunately, this type of medicine is representative of Neanderthal mentality. The comprehensive testing done never once focused on potential underlying causes. If the hospital did uncover the underlying causes, they would have to admit that childhood vaccines are dangerous and another adverse report would have to be submitted to the Centers for Disease Control and Prevention.

The video testimonial says it all. An integrated approach that defines the cause(s) plus using natural remedies is the most efficacious and noninvasive way to treat humans, especially toddlers. I strongly recommend that all parents of young children read two of Dr. Robert S. Mendelsohn's books, *Confession of a Medical*

Heretic and *Ritual Mutilations*. Dr. Mendelsohn was a medical pediatrician who blew the whistle on the medical establishment. One mother's response was "I read this book when my children were small, and I think it may have saved their lives."

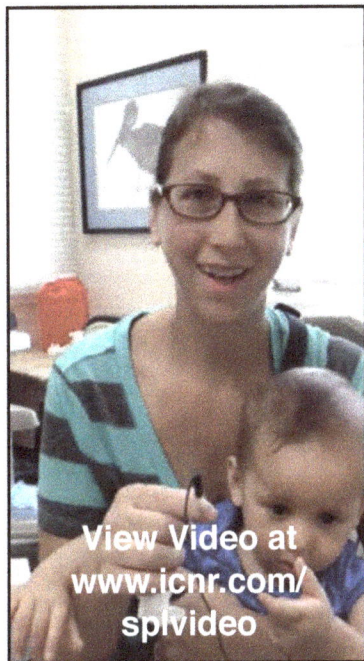

View Video at
www.icnr.com/
splvideo

Conclusion: The exorbitant amount of money paid by the insurance company in reality did not bring any beneficial return to the little toddler or his parents.

Medical Disclaimer: When you walk into the "Ivory Tower" (hospital), do not think for one minute that the professional staff really know what they are doing.

I strongly recommend that all parents faced with the vaccination decision peruse the National Vaccine Information Center site (www.nvic.org). Armed with their information, you will be able to make a more informed decision.

It is bad enough to give vaccines to infants, but now Big Pharma is pushing flu shots on pregnant women to "protect" the unborn from potential damage. In my opinion, this is tantamount to child abuse and is criminal. The blood-brain barrier of a baby does not fully mature until 18 months after birth. Whatever toxins introduced into the mother will find their way into the fetus' organs, especially the brain. Don't be intimidated by the medical establishment. Get proactive and do your research. The best defense is being armed with knowledge. Damaging an unborn baby will become a lifetime of heartache.

Research on ten newborn babies conducted by the Environmental Working Group (EWG) found on average 287 chemicals in their blood drawn from their placentas at birth. The EWG spent $50,000 on each child to analyze his or her blood. Knowing that your child has approximately 287 chemicals in his or her blood at birth, does it make any sense to give the child a hepatitis B shot two days after it is born. Their immune system has not had a chance to mature.

The Mystery of Bipolar Disorder Uncovered

The following letter was provided by one of my patients after reversing his bipolar problem.

"I wanted to write a letter conveying my appreciation for your guidance and direction in helping me extract the mercury from my body, especially my thyroid and brain. Your expertise has enabled me to be completely free of any medications I was on to stabilize my bipolar condition. In other words, I believe I am cured.

I have suffered since 1976 from a bipolar disorder which was then called manic depression. I was on a high maintenance level of lithium carbonate. Later, upon other hospital visits, the addition of Depakote and Zoloft completed my medication cocktail. Presently, I have been free and clear of any symptoms and have been off the medications for over a year. Since my father was a dentist from the time I was a young boy he had filled my cavities with mercury, silver fillings.

Until recently, I was unaware that mercury was the malleable substrate that gave the filling its pliability and its durability. I found to my amazement that the acids from the body broke down the mercury/silver composite, allowing the majority of the fillings 'makeup—mercury—to break down and thus leach into my body. Since the thyroid is below the jaw and the brain is directly above the mouth, the mercury did not have to travel far to cause problems.

The thyroid enables the one pole of the bipolar—depression—to occur when infused with the liquid mercury. As simplistically as I understand the ramifications of mercury poisoning, the brain easily short circuits as a direct result of degeneration of brain cells. Mercury vapors travel easily into the body during the chewing process. In addition, mercury has been well documented to leak out of mercury fillings 24/7, and especially if one drinks hot fluids like coffee or tea. Understanding the damaging effects of mercury gave me more insight into the nature of my bipolar disorder. It also helped me understand why I acted the way I did for so many years. The fact that I learned of the underlying cause of my bipolar condition enabled me to eradicate the problem.

Dr. Smith, you have helped me get off the maintenance program of the medication nightmare the psychologists had me on for so many years. I cannot express my gratitude enough. The actual feeling of knowing that I have been cured from this bipolar disorder and the anxiety that resulted from it is quite a relief. I suffered from the time I was sixteen, although diagnosed at nineteen years of age, up until I was forty-four. This all came about because of mercury poisoning from the fillings that were implanted by my dad my dentist. My father learned a heart-wrenching lesson and has discontinued the use of mercury in his practice.

I thank you from the bottom of my soul,

Reverend H.S.

The following chart of symptoms of mercury toxicity is provided to educate people of the potential dangers of this American Dental Association approved material:

Symptoms of Mercury Toxicity

If a person has 7 or more of these symptoms, there is a significantly increased possibility that mercury toxicity is a major contributing factor.

· **CENTRAL NERVOUS SYSTEM**
· Irritability
· Anxiety/nervousness, often with difficulty breathing
· Restlessness
· Exaggerated response to stimulation
· Fearfulness
· Emotional instability
- Lack of self-control
- Fits of anger, with violent, irrational behavior
· Loss of self-confidence
· Indecision
· Shyness or timidity, being easily embarrassed
· Loss of memory
· Inability to concentrate
· Lethargy, drowsiness
· Insomnia
· Mental depression, despondency
· Withdrawal
· Suicidal tendencies
· Manic-depression
· Numbness and tingling of hands, feet, fingers, toes, or lips
· Muscle weakness progressing to paralysis
· Ataxia
· Tremors/trembling of hands, feet, lips, eyelids, or tongue
· Incoordination
· Myoneural transmission failure resembling Myasthenia gravis
· Multiple sclerosis

· **GASTROINTESTINAL EFFECTS**
· Food sensitivities, especially to milk and eggs
· Abdominal cramps, colitis, diverticulitis, or other G.I. complaints
· Chronic diarrhea/constipation

· **CARDIOVASCULAR EFFECTS**
· Abnormal heart rhythm

- Characteristic findings on EKG
- Abnormal changes in the S-T segment and/or lower
- Broadened P wave
- Unexplained elevated serum triglycerides
- Unexplained elevated cholesterol
- Abnormal blood pressure, either high or low

- **IMMUNOLOGIC**
- Repeated infections
- Viral and fungal
- Myobacterial
- *Candida* and other yeast infections
- Cancer
- Autoimmune disorders
- Arthritis
- Lupis erythematosus (LE)
- Multiple sclerosis (MS)
- Scleroderma
- Amyolateral sclerosis (ALS)
- Hypothyroidism

- **HEAD, NECK, ORAL CAVITY DISORDERS**
- Bleeding gums
- Alveolar bone loss
- Loosening of teeth
- Excessive salivation
- Foul breath
- Metallic taste
- Burning sensation, with tingling of lips, face
- Tissue pigmentation (amalgam tattoo of gums)
- Leukoplakia
- Stomatitis
- Ulceration of gingiva, palate, tongue
- Dizziness/acute, chronic vertigo
- Ringing in ears
- Hearing difficulties
- Speech and visual impairment
- Glaucoma
- Restricted, dim vision

- **SYSTEMIC EFFECTS**
- Chronic headaches
- Allergies
- Severe dermatitis
- Unexplained reactivity
- Thyroid disturbance
- Subnormal body temperature
- Cold, clammy skin, especially hands and feet
- Excessive perspiration, with frequent night sweats
- Unexplained sensory symptoms, including pain
- Unexplained numbness or burning sensations
- Unexplained anemia
- G-6-PD deficiency
- Chronic kidney disease
  - Nephrotic syndrome
  - Receiving renal dialysis
  - Kidney infection
- Adrenal disease
- General fatigue
- Loss of appetite, with or without weight loss
- Loss of weight
- Hypoglycemia

Eight Years of Chronic Pain Caused by Third Molar Extractions

Most people are walking time bombs and don't even know it. Adam was a perfect example. He followed the advice of his dentist and had his wisdom teeth removed. After several months, his pain symptoms started appearing. He even developed a severe clenching habit. His journey took him to Harvard School of Dentistry, numerous oral surgeons, dentists, chiropractors, neurologists, and other health care practitioners in hopes of resolving his chronic neck, middle, and low back pain. Unfortunately, none of the therapies worked. In addition to the fact that the healthcare practitioners who evaluated Adam did not know what to look for, they treated him with minimal respect. Because of their lack of knowledge, they tried to shift the causation by telling Adam that it was all in his head. These practitioners were absolutely correct, but they didn't have a clue as to what to look for.

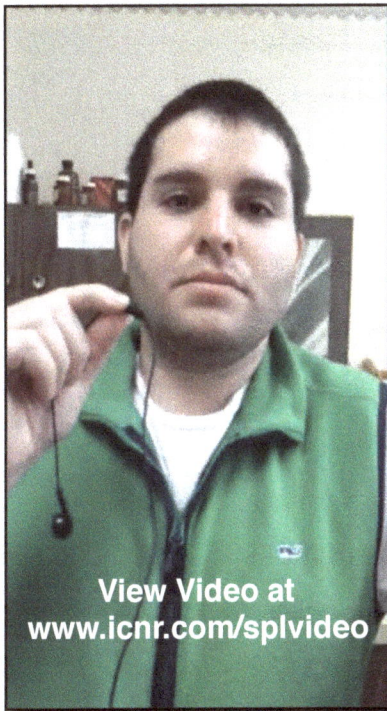

The major missing link in Adam's pain puzzle was the fact that the extraction of his wisdom teeth caused a direct distortion of his cranial motion. This iatrogenically caused distortion placed a pull in his dural membrane system that extended down to his sacrum. Adam also had a complicating factor that helped to perpetuate his pain pattern. He had a slight malocclusion, that caused an abnormal contact on his lower left second molar tooth. The excess force on an incline of his second molar was causing his temporal bones to rotate out of alignment. This distortion caused a twisting of his body, with resultant muscle pain. Since functional anatomy is not part of the routine curriculum in dental or medical schools, this information is unknown to most conventional dentists and medical doctors. Because of their ignorance, Adam experienced varying degrees of ridicule from the uninformed doctors.

View Video at www.icnr.com/splvideo

After evaluating Adam's skull for specific cranial distortions, it was evident to me that the removal of his wisdom teeth was the basis for his problem. A comprehensive cranial adjustment was done to correct the misalignment. Following the adjustment, the offending occlusal or tooth interference was removed. Adam immediately experienced a reduction of 99% of his pain.

The bite correction helped stabilize his cranium and allowed his muscles to realign and remain pain-free.

What is Cranial Manipulation and Why Is it so Important?

The human skull is made up of 28 bones. These bony plates are connected by sutures. The sutures are expansion-contraction joints that permit micromotion between the plates. Traumas like whiplash, falls, blows to the head, plus iatrogenic causes from dental procedures like straightening teeth, having a tooth filled, having a crown or implant placed, and extractions all have one thing in common: they all have the potential to cause distortions to the alignment of the cranial bones. Misalignment of the 28 bones of the skull will directly affect the flow of cerebrospinal fluid (CSF) around the brain and create neurologic distortions in the central and autonomic nervous systems (sympathetic [gas pedal] and parasympathetic [brakes]).

Cranial manipulation was discovered in the 1920s by Nephi Cottam, D.C. and refined through the years by such pioneers as Andrew Taylor Still, D.O., William G. Sutherland, D.O., Harold Magoun, D.O., John Upledger, D.O., Major B. DeJarnette, D.C., Marc Pick, D.C., Viola Fryman, D.O., George Goodhardt, D.C., and Cleo A. Bludworth, D.C., to name a few of the innovators of this speciality. Using gentle pressures, a skilled practitioner can diagnose and then realign or reset the bones.

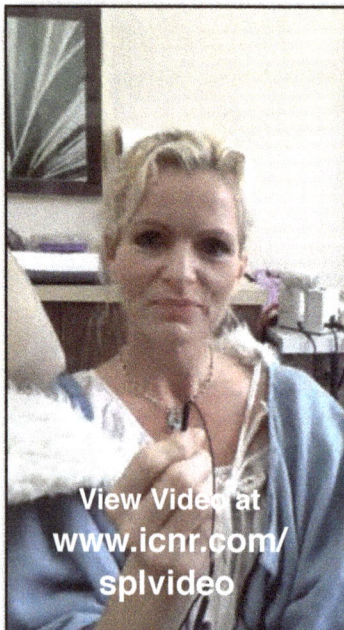

View Video at www.icnr.com/splvideo

Dysfunction of the body has many underlying causes however, cranial distortions represent one area that is often overlooked by most physicians. Removing the distortions will have a major impact on restoring the feeling of well being. Cranial correction removes a major stressor from the brain, spine, and pelvis. Following a cranial manipulation session, patients often remark that they feel more relaxed, their occlusion (bite) feels more comfortable when their teeth touch, their eyesight is clearer, their mental fog lifts, and many of their pains (neck, shoulders, arms, hands, lower back) disappear. Re-establishing CSF flow reactivates the brain, muscles, cognitive function, and much more, allowing the whole system to feel more normal.

The following testimonial was unsolicited from a recent patient.

"Just wanted to drop a quick note to say that it was a pleasure to meet with you (and Rebecca). I am not sure what it is, but I felt more refreshed when I woke up this morning. Believe this is a start and I began taking the supplements this morning. Can't imagine what state I will be after a few months! Look forward to staying on your recommended path towards recovery and thank you for your service. Have a good weekend! — Best,—John—K."

Twenty-One Years and Nine Months Post-Concussion Symptoms Resolved in One Treatment

Andrew Adams had suffered chronic severe headaches since December of 1995. While at a college hockey game, he was hit on the top of his head by a 65 pound panel of glass that was knocked loose, by two players that collided, at rink side. Andrew was incapacitated and unable to work for four months. In addition to the 24/7 headaches, he would experience excruciating head pain when the weather changed. Andrew was treated by numerous headache/pain centers including Mayo Clinic, Johns Hopkins, U. of Pennsylvania with no lasting results. All pain medications, botox, and Imitrex injections did not resolve his headaches. On Monday, August 14, 2017, Andrew was examined in my office. He was diagnosed with a trauma-induced cranial distortion that was the direct result of his 1995 incident.

Treatment consisted of a comprehensive cranial adjustment. The process took one hour. At the end of the adjustment session, Andrew stated that his headaches of twenty-one years and nine months' duration had resolved. On August 21, 2017, exactly one week later, Andrew was seen in my office. Andrew stated that he had been headache-free since the initial adjustment. In addition, several storms had occurred during the one-week post-treatment period, and Andrew stated that he had not experienced any headaches from the barometric pressure change. Of interest, Andrew also stated that all his friends had told him that he looked younger and more at peace since his treatment.

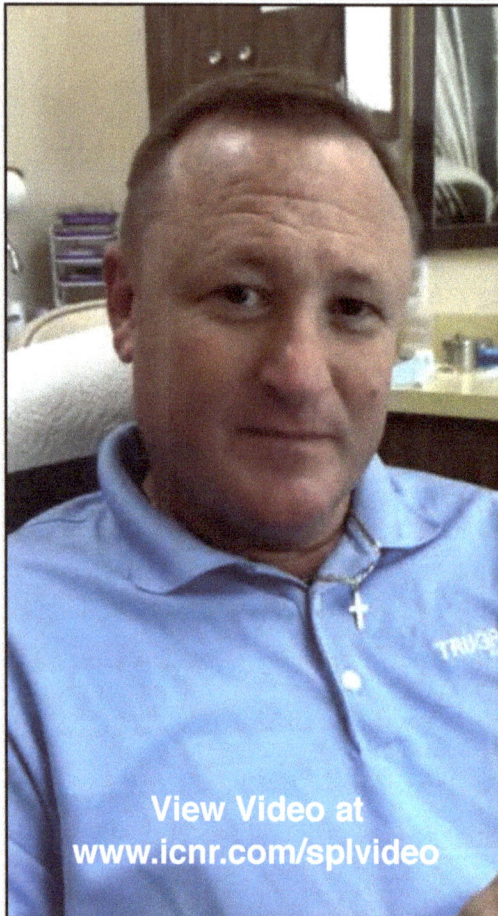

View Video at www.icnr.com/splvideo

Concussion is a complex medical issue. The sequelae go beyond the swelling, bruising, bleeding, and possible damage to the brain tissue. Doctor Smith, who has been a pioneer in the field of dental cranial distortions, has recognized that there is a structural component to concussion that has not been previously diagnosed.

The key component to head trauma is the fact that the basic motion of the skull becomes reversed, hampering the flow of CSF and increased tension in the intra cranial dural membrane system. The latter issue is the cause of the constant pain and the former, is the cause of distorted skull motion, and is responsible for the mental fog, poor memory, fatigue and other symptoms related to concussion.

Twenty Years of Migraine Headaches Resolved with One Cranial Adjustment

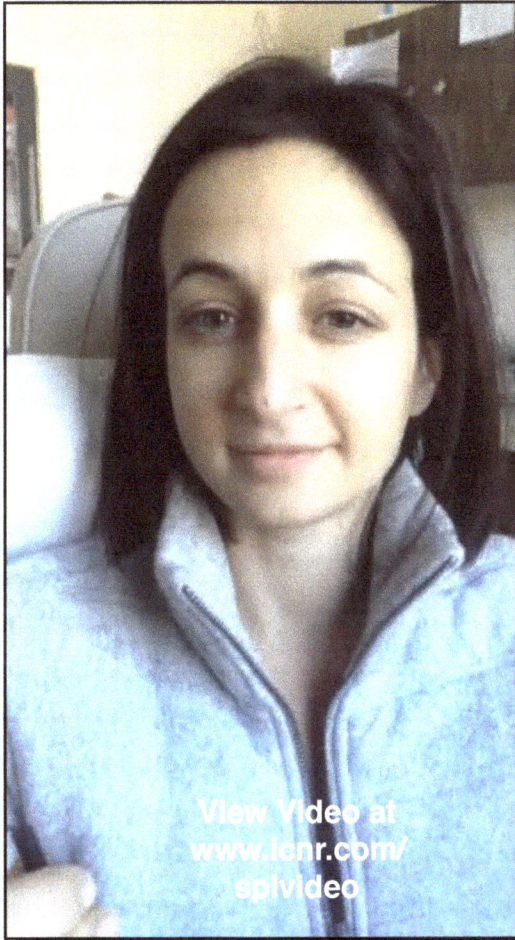

Danielle had suffered severe migraine headaches for the last 20 years. Also, alcohol would trigger her migraines. Danielle had a medical history (from several automobile accidents) of three whiplash injuries and two concussions as a child. She was prescribed many drugs for pain, which brought only temporary relief.

Evaluation revealed several major cranial bone distortions, which had never been diagnosed, and several factors involving heavy metal contamination and nutritional deficiencies. In December of 2014, the patient flew in from Tobago, Trinidad, and received treatment from me consisting of a cranial adjustment and a nutritional program to restore existing imbalances and to achieve liver detoxification to remove existing contaminants. Her 20 years of migraine headaches were totally eliminated in one treatment.

In addition, after six weeks on nutritional supplements to detox her liver, the alcohol trigger totally resolved. Unfortunately, conventional medicine has no knowledge of this "advanced technology".

Six Years of Post-Whiplash Injuries Resolved in One-Half Hour

Doctor Tran had been in a severe motor vehicle accident 20 years ago. She was not wearing a seat belt in the vehicle, and she incurred multiple traumas from the movement of a table that was being transported. Six years ago, Dr. Tran developed constant numbness down her left arm accompanied by tingling. She also developed a painful trigger point in her left trapezius muscle in her rear shoulder area. Because of the pain she was unable to sleep through the night and to sleep on her left side due to the pain. In addition, Doctor Tran suffered stomach pains and heartburn-like symptoms that would also waken her from sleep.

Medically, Dr. Tran had undergone computed tomographic scans to assess brain injuries, but nothing had shown up. She also underwent osteopathic evaluation and treatment with no lasting results. Traditional medicine ran the full gamut of testing and had nothing else to offer with the exception of drug management of the pain, which she refused.

While attending Dr. Smith's January 2017 seminar in Toronto, Dr. Tran was evaluated for cranial distortions. Specific trauma-induced cranial lesions were found. Doctor Smith provided a full cranial adjustment, which resulted in an immediate disappearance of all her symptoms. Even though cranial manipulation was developed in the 1930s, the majority of health care practitioners are unaware of the far-reaching positive effects this noninvasive therapy has to offer.

Post-Whiplash Sequelae of Eight Months Resolved in One Treatment

Doctor Tey was hospitalized for post-whiplash sequelae involving pain, burning, and numbness from cervical vertebrae two to seven and down the left arm. MRIs,

CT scans, physical therapy, and chiropractic treatment were unable to resolve her symptoms for eight months. The hospital physicians gave a diagnosis of possible stroke. After Dr. Smith evaluated the patient's cranium, a diagnosis was made of torsions and asynchronous motion. Dr. Smith's treatment involved a cranial adjustment to remove the cranial dural membrane tension and correct the asynchronous motion. Immediately following the adjustment, the patient's burning, pain, and numbness totally disappeared. The following day the patient stated that she slept through the night for the first time in eight months with the need for sleeping pills.

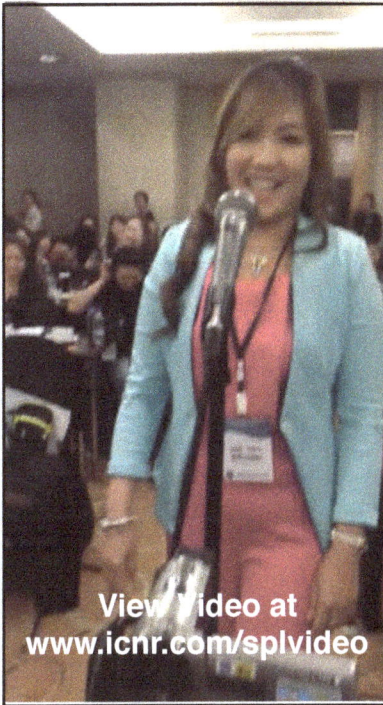

View Video at www.icnr.com/splvideo

One and a Half Years' Post-Whiplash Pain Resolved

Ron Goldberg was in a car accident in 2008. For 18 months, he suffered pain down the left side of his body plus distortion of vision. Ron tried many different forms of therapy, including acupuncture, chiropractic and physical therapy — none of which addressed the underlying cause. Ron's cranial motion was traumatized, which resulted in an asynchronous motion of his skull bones. Tightening of the dural membrane tensioned the spinal nerves down the entire length of his spine. Applied therapies failed to resolve this causative tension, and his pain persisted. Dr. Smith's treatment involved cranial manipulation, which resynchronized his skull

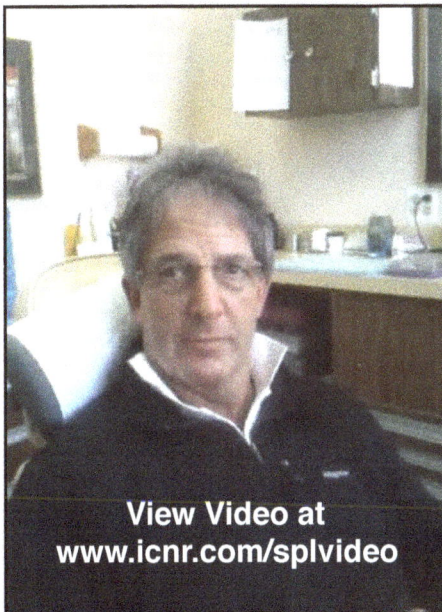

motion back to factory default. Immediately following correction, Ron's 18 months of pain totally disappeared and he stated that his vision improved by 60 percent.

Post-Whiplash Pain

Someone once stated that a genius is someone who recognizes the obvious. Through my 50 years of post-graduate training, I have had the good fortune of studying with a handful of geniuses who taught me basic concepts of how the human body really works. My contribution was the ability to integrate these various concepts into a comprehensive treatment approach.

Every structure must have a stable foundation. The human body is no different. One key area that is overlooked by 99.9% of practitioners is the functional motion of the human skull. There is a natural rhythm that governs its motion. A traumatic accident such as a whiplash injury, a fall on the ice, or even a tooth extraction often disrupts this rhythm. When this occurs, tension is dramatically increased along the entire dural membrane system that extends from around the brain, through the base of the skull, attaches to the upper three cervical vertebrae, and then travels down to its final attachment at the second sacral tubercle. This is why it is referred to as the cranial sacral system. When the neck muscles get injured from microtrauma from a motor vehicle or similar incident, the dural membrane tension directly affects the entire nervous system. Often patients exhibit pain patterns down one half of the body that do not respond to conventional therapies. The reason is simple. The underlying cause is not being corrected. The following two video case testimonials reinforce this basic concept.

Fifteen-Year Migraine Headaches Resolved

Ever since Marta was 16-years-old, she had been plagued by migraine headaches. This malady derailed her aspirations of becoming a professional dancer. Many avenues of medical treatments were pursued, with no positive results. Marta's husband, a dentist, was attending one of Dr. Smith's seminars. As part of the hands-on demonstrations, Marta was examined for potential sources of her migraine headaches. Marta's primary core issue was misalignment of her skull bones. Treatment in the form of a gentle cranial adjustment was performed on that day in April of 2013. Following that one treatment in April, Marta has not experienced any migraine headaches. Besides the disappearance of her migraine headaches, her posture dramatically improved. Her husband stated that previously whenever Marta rode her motorcycle, her body would lean to one side. Following the cranial alignment, Marta was able to sit straight on her cycle.

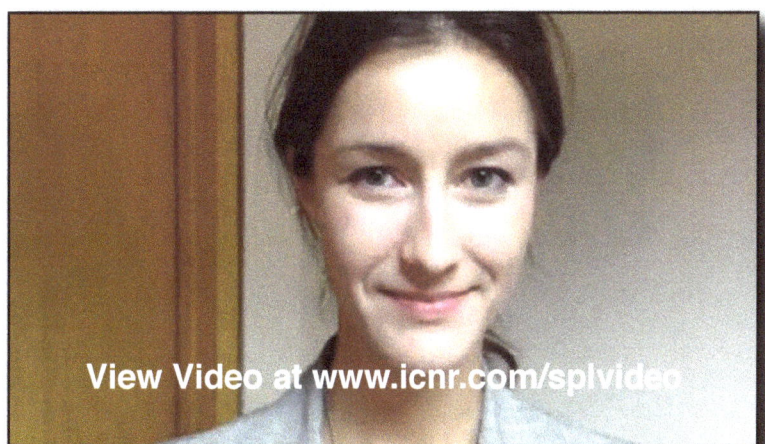

View Video at www.icnr.com/splvideo

Footnote: Cranial misalignment is a major factor in many chronic pain issues. Unfortunately, most health care professionals do not possess the diagnostic and treatment skills to uncover cranial misalignment or correct it if they are present. It is a sad commentary that cranial therapy, which originated back in the 1930's, has not become more mainstream.

Concussion Revisited: Sixteen Years Post-Concussion Syndrome Resolved in 1.5 Hours

Ziyi Zhu, a 22-year-old Chinese boy, had suffered post-concussion symptoms since he was six years old, when he was knocked unconscious from a fall. Headaches, mental fog, his head feeling heavy, pressure in the back of the head, neck pain, and a feeling of fatigue had plagued Ziyi for the past 16 years.

Chapter Four - Cranial Complex

The patient stated that he had seen 100 doctors in combination for treatment and/or consultation. Both traditional and Chinese medicine were unable to solve his problems. Ziyi found my website, www.icnr.com, and found that symptoms were similar to those presented in case study #64 (ten years of neck and lower back pain due to faulty orthodontics). After a number of e-mail correspondences, Ziyi decided to fly in from China for evaluation and treatment. It was ultimately found that the original concussion had created cranial distortions that were overlaid by additional distortions resulting from orthodontic treatment had exacerbated his original symptoms.

A comprehensive cranial examination was performed on June 29, 2017. Clinically, Ziyi presented with a full reversed motion of the base of his skull overlaid with other individual cranial bone distortions. He was then treated with gentle cranial manipulation and scalar energy technology (Theraphi). In an hour and a half, Ziyi's symptoms of mental fog, heavy head, neck pain, pressure in the back of his head, and feeling of fatigue totally resolved. He stated that he experienced a wonderful sense of calm following treatment.

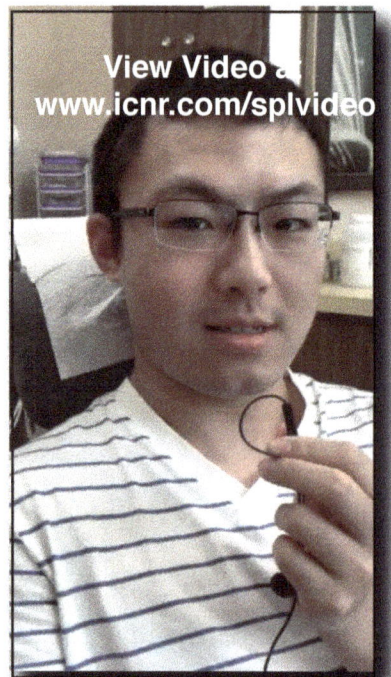

View Video at www.icnr.com/splvideo

Chapter Four - Cranial Complex

For too long post-concussion patients have suffered needlessly because the healthcare industry is not aware of cranial manipulation technology. Re-establishing balance of the cranial motion helps restore normal brain function. This aspect is another major piece of the concussion puzzle that still eludes physicians. This last case just like the others presented in this book, drive home the message, that practitioners must get back to basics.

As a pioneer in the field of post-concussion treatment, I have developed five simple cranial indicators that once learned can determine in 30 seconds the three dimensional distortions of the skull. No CT scan, magnetic resonance imaging, or x-ray system can give the practitioner this information. It is extremely important that all healthcare practitioners learn this system. Without it patients are getting short changed and his or her examinations are incomplete. Patients must get proactive and demand that their practitioner raise his skill levels to include a comprehensive cranial evaluation when they present with a history of concussion, whiplash injury, and chronic symptoms such as those mentioned above.

The Cranial Complex is one major area in which most healthcare practitioners are lacking knowledge of. Most professional schools do not teach this specialty during their four-year program. The reason it is not taught is simple. There is too much basic information that must be learned, plus the concepts of the cranial complex are too sophisticated to grasp. In reality, it takes about eight to ten years of practice and post-graduate seminars before a practitioner is capable of mastering this specialty.

"The whole art of medicine is in observation…. The physician can only see what he was trained to see."

William Osler

Chapter Five: Dental Complex

Stomatognathic System - Dental Complex

The thirty-two teeth that make up the dentition represent a complex circuit breaker system that relates to specific organs, muscles, vertebra, and nervous system. Embryologically the front teeth, canines, laterals, and incisors all develop from the neural tube, which give rise to the sympathetic part of your nervous system. The sympathetic part of your nervous system acts like the gas pedal on your car. It is essential for your fight-or-flight mechanism of survival. Sympathetic stimulation causes your heart to race, blood vessels to constrict, your mouth to become dry, decrease in the motility of your digestive system, and dilate both your pupils and pulmonary bronchioles.

The posterior teeth, bicuspids and molars develop embryologically from the neural crest cells which give rise to the parasympathetic part of your nervous system. When stimulated the parasympathetic nervous system slows the heart, dilates the blood vessels, increases salivation, increases peristaltic motion of the intestines, constricts both the pupils and pulmonary bronchioles.

Teeth Whole Body Connection

In the 1950s, Dr. Reinhold Voll, an East German medical doctor and engineer, was the first researcher to link the teeth to the various parts of the body. Interestingly when a tooth becomes injured by decay, infection or hyper occlusion (heavy bite), the nervous system of that tooth can directly affect specific muscles, organs, and vertebra associated with that tooth. In essence, having a bad bite (malocclusion), a restored filling that is too high, a filling that is too low, or a toxic filling material like mercury can directly cause pain in associated structures. A case in point was a patient of mine whose wife I was treating for severe cranial distortions, keep insisting that her husband let me examine his bite. For eight years Robert endured low back pain. The low back pain initiated immediately after his dentist cemented in a crown on his lower right second molar. Evaluation determined that a minor bite interference existed on the distal lingual cusp of the crown as noted by the red line on the photograph.

Removal of the minor interference immediately resolved the eight years of low back pain. That incident occurred in 2000 and the patient has never had a recurrence.

Ten Years of Facial, Neck, and Lower Back Pain Due to Faulty Orthodontics

The maxilla or upper jaw represents the anterior two thirds of the base of the cranium. It represents the foundation of the human skull. When this anatomical component is violated it can wreak havoc on the rest of the body. Beverly M. was referred to my office in 2004 for evaluation and treatment for sever facial pain, difficulty talking, neck and shoulder pain, TMJ pain, chronic headaches, fatigue, and inability to sleep through the night because of the pain. Beverly's symptoms all started after she completed conventional orthodontic treatment that was finalized in 1994. During the ten years before she ended up on my doorstep, Beverly was examined by fifty doctors, with no resolution to her symptoms.

Conventional orthodontic treatment had compressed her maxilla and created a transverse tilt of her maxilla that was high on the right side. Within 24 hours of inserting and properly adjusting an ALF (Advanced Lightwire Functional Appliance) to help correct her cranial distortions that were iatrogenically created by the faulty orthodontics, Beverly experienced dramatic reduction in her facial pain. After two years of expansion and correction of the alignment of her teeth and her maxilla and mandible, Beverly was completely pain free. In addition, she also had mercury

BEVERLY MARSH

ALF placed and adjusted to balance the four cranial indicators. Pain greatly reduced within 24 hours.

Pre-Tx

24 hours post ALF insertion

toxicity that contributed to many of her symptoms. A detoxification program was instituted to alleviate the problem. The enclosed photos document the dramatic change that resulted from the expansion process. Unfortunately, most dentists have no clue that the cranial bones move and distort when faulty orthodontic procedures are used to move the teeth. If ISIS would learn the techniques of modern orthodontics they would be infinitely more efficient in inflicting pain to their captures.

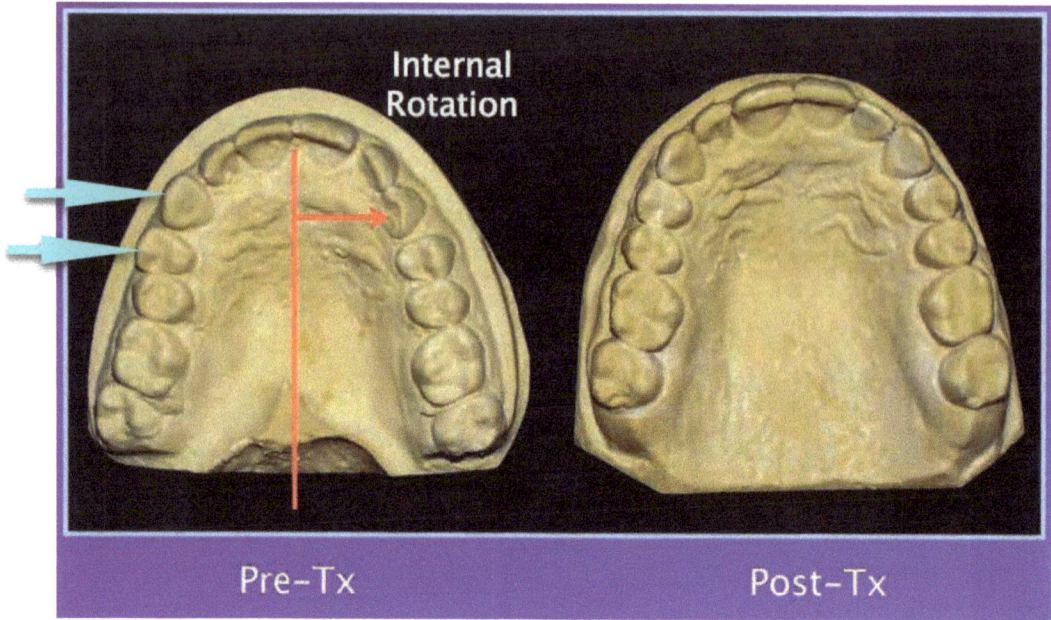

Internal
Rotation

Pre-Tx   Post-Tx

Beverly's cranial base was expanded and corrected 3-dimensionally. The red arrow depicts the reduce width of the left half of the palate which is narrower than the right half. The decreased space represents an internal rotation of the left half of the maxilla. In addition, her maxilla was torqued or rotated clockwise as noted by the position of the right canine and bicuspid teeth.

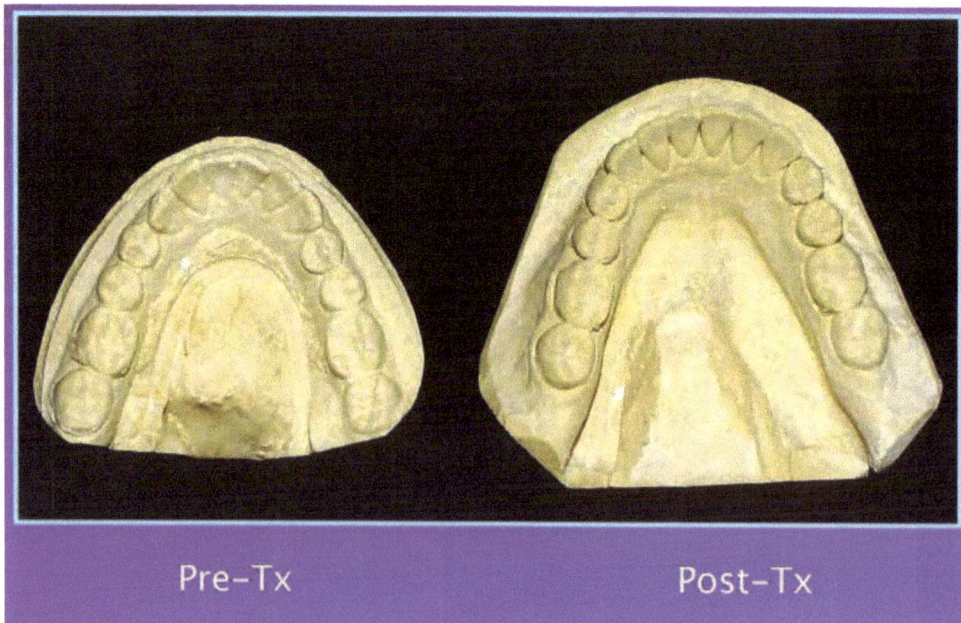

Pre-Tx   Post-Tx

Beverly's mandibular arch was expanded to fit the maxillary template, which also provided more space for her tongue.

Chapter Five: Dental Complex

Ten Years of Headaches, Neck and Lower Back Pain Due to Faulty Orthodontics

University trained orthodontists focus primarily on straightening the teeth and providing a pretty smile. The only caveat to this approach is that they know not what they do. If you don't believe me just ask your orthodontist what direct affect the braces have on the cranium. Then watch for the puzzled look on his or here face.

This case study is a perfect example of what I have been saying for years. Ian Hedley was treated by an orthodontist who had a master degree in orthodontics. Four bicuspid teeth were extracted and retraction orthodontics applied. At age 14, Ian was an excellent athlete and great student. Once his bicuspid teeth were removed and the braces applied, Ian literally fell apart. Chronic neck and lower back pain coupled with chronic fatigue and mental fog set in. For fourteen years, Ian literally flew around the globe looking for answers. Three orthodontists later Ian landed on my doorstep. The problem was staring every one right in their face but they could not see it. The original orthodontist with the master degree had

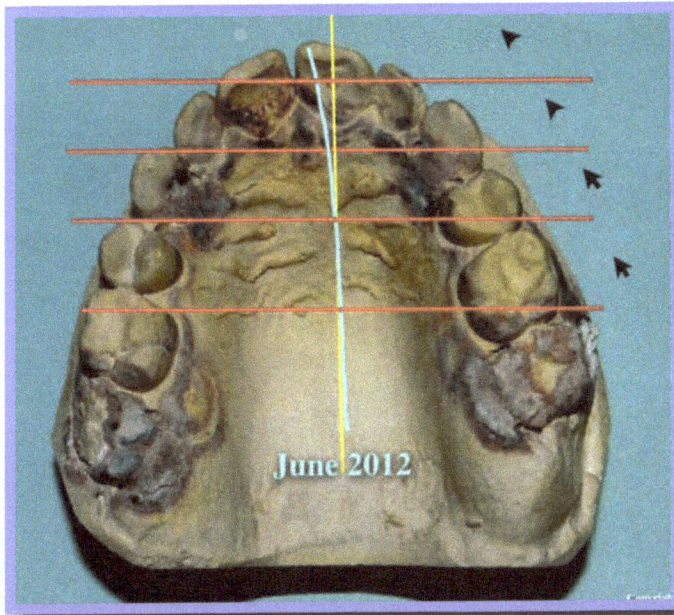

June 2012

rotated Ian's maxilla counterclockwise, which in turn twisted his dural membrane down to his sacrum. Using Dr. Smith's Cranial Indicator System would have prevented this tragedy and needless suffering from occurring.

Resolution of the case was by design. The Cranial Indicators developed by Dr. Smith provide the only noninvasive diagnostic approach for monitoring treatment progress. No matter what orthodontic technique being used if

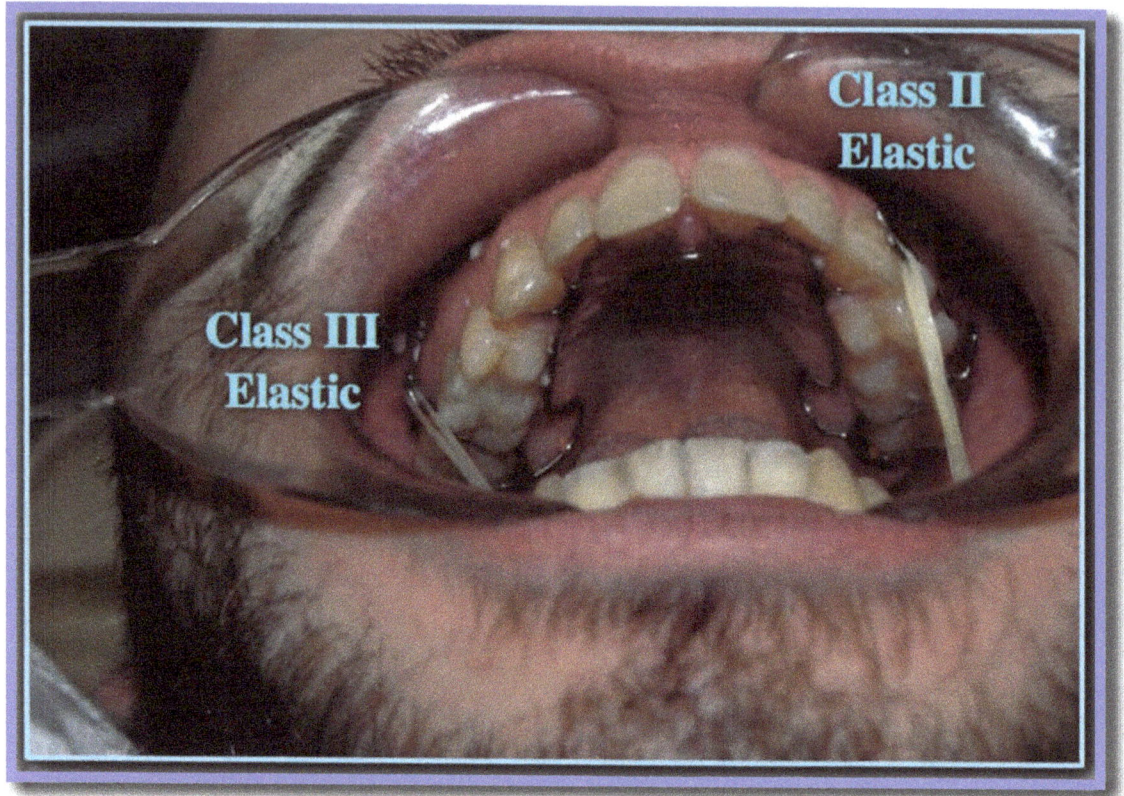

the orthodontist is not monitoring the direct effects of his or her treatment on your cranial bone alignment, you may be in for the surprise of your life.

Einstein defined insanity as "doing the same thing over again and expecting a different result."

Correcting Ian's twisted maxilla (palate) and dural membrane system required use of the ALF appliance in conjunction with specially placed elastics. Without the use of Dr. Smith's Cranial Indicators it is virtually impossible to monitor the cranial bone changes during treatment. The indicators also provide an endpoint to treatment.

As a result of correcting Ian's cranial distortions, Ian got his life back. He was able to travel to Australia, a 24-hour flight, without back pain. He also was able to play golf again without any pain. Unfortunately, the orthodontic community has no clue regarding the interrelationship of the teeth to the cranium, spine, and pelvis.

View Video at
www.icnr.com/splinters

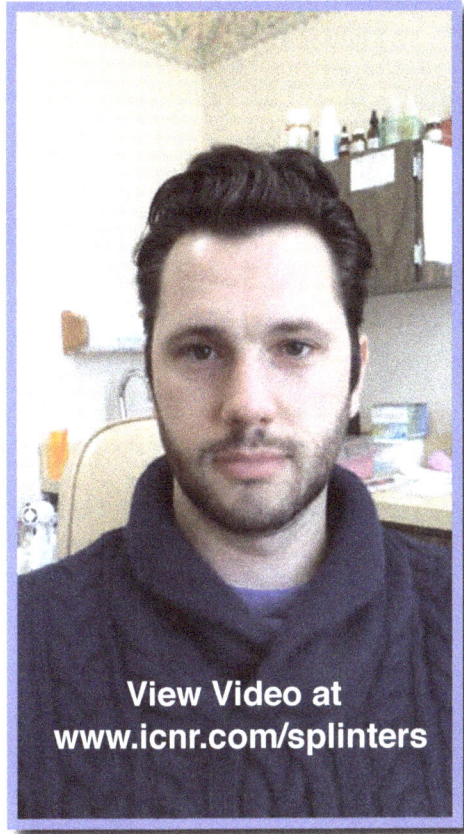

Completed Case

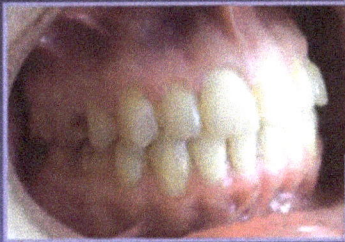

The key to successful Tx was defining the counterclockwise rotation of the maxillae.

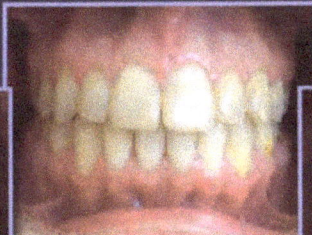

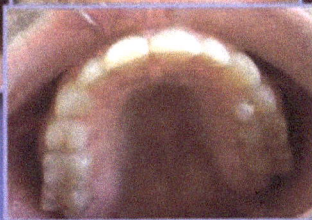

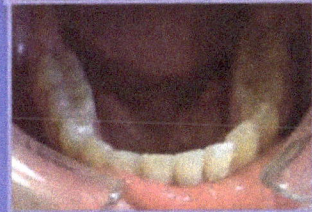

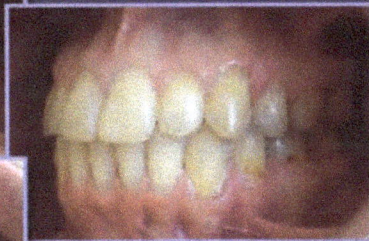

It is more important to achieve occlusal cranial balance than establishing a class I molar relationship or getting the mid-lines straight!

Copyright Gerald H. Smith, DDS 2016

Eight Years of Chronic Pain Due to Third Molar Extractions

Most people are walking time bombs and don't even know it. Adam was a perfect example. He followed the advice of his dentist and had his wisdom teeth removed. After several months his pain symptoms started appearing. He even developed a sever clenching habit. His journey took him to Harvard School of Dentistry and numerous oral surgeons, dentists, chiropractors, neurologists and other health care practitioners in hopes of resolving his chronic neck and middle and lower back pain. Unfortunately, none of the therapies worked.

The major missing link in Adam's pain puzzle was the fact that the extraction of his wisdom teeth caused a direct distortion to his cranial motion. This iatrogenic caused distortion placed a pull in his dural membrane system that extended down to his sacrum. Adam also had a complicating factor which helped to perpetuate his pain pattern. He had a slight malocclusion which caused an abnormal contact on his lower left second molar. The excess force on an incline plane of his second molar was causing his temporal bones to rotate out of alignment. This distortion caused a twisting of his body with resultant muscle pain. Since functional anatomy is not part of the standard curriculum in dental or medical schools, this information is unknown to most conventional dentists and medical doctors. Because of their ignorance, Adam experienced varying degrees of ridicule from the uninformed doctors of higher learning.

After evaluating Adam's skull for specific cranial distortions, it was evident to me that the removal of his wisdom teeth was the basis for his problem. A comprehensive cranial adjustment was done to correct the misalignment. Following the adjustment, the offending occlusal or tooth interference was removed. Adam immediately experienced a reduction of 99% of his pain.

The bite correction helped stabilize his cranium and allow his muscles to realign and remain pain free.

View Video at
www.icnr.com/splinters

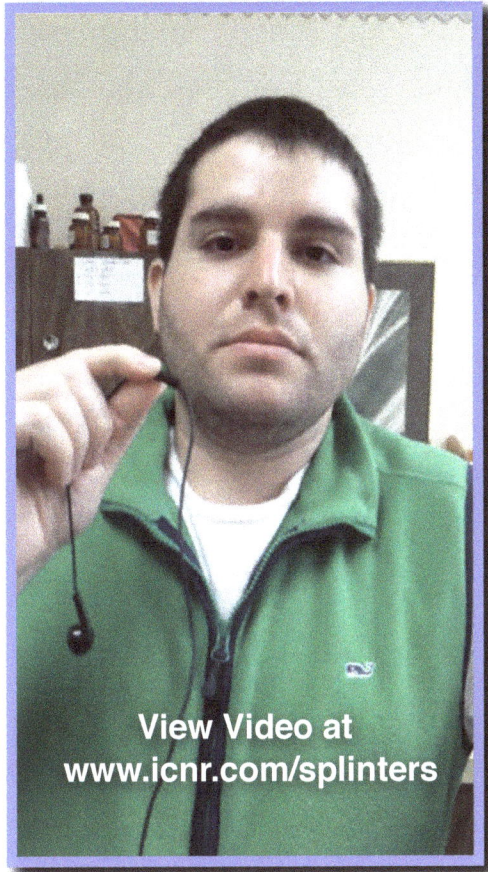

Tooth Extraction/Herpes Zoster (Shingles) Connection

The unrelenting pain of chronic shingles can easily ruin one's quality of life and even drive one to thoughts of suicide. Traditional medical concepts relating to shingles still focuses on antiquated allopathic myths that shingles cannot be cured. Present day medicine gives patients little hope of resolving their pain while embracing the belief that symptomatic relief is still the gold standard of treatment.

New technology based on quantum physics is now available to help practitioners quickly diagnose and effectively treat herpes zoster (shingles). There is no need for patients to continue to suffer. The causative agent is a virus and viruses can be effectively treated with biofrequencies and basic nutritional therapy. There are specific minerals, vitamins, herbs and homeopathics that help suppress the virus within the cells. Other nutrients are effective in boosting the patient's immune system to help keep the virus under control. An integrated, noninvasive approach is extremely effective in bringing relief to chronic shingles sufferers.

A case in point is a young chiropractor who suffered severe left side facial, nose, maxillary sinus, eye and ear pain for over a year. The pain started immediately after the local anesthetic wore off after an oral surgeon removed an impacted upper left third molar. For a little over one year this patient experienced unrelenting pain. This patient became desperate when she started to loose the sight of her left eye and hearing in her left ear. Not one of the many specialists that were visited was able to make a definitive diagnosis. Within five minutes of examining the patient, a diagnosis of shingles in the extraction site was made and treatment initiated. Within one hour of quantum therapy, the patient reported an 80% reduction in pain after she had endured severe pain for a little over one year.

The newer quantum technology is incredibly effective, safe, and noninvasive.

Facial Pain / Dental Connection

JM suffered with facial pain for twenty-two years despite extensive medical, dental, chiropractic evaluations and even surgical intervention. JM's saga began in her twenties, when she had seventeen crowns fabricated to restore her posterior teeth. The dentist who performed the restorations was competent from a mechanical perspective, that is, the anatomical crown forms, porcelain shade and marginal fit all fell within the standard of care as defined by the dental schools. Unfortunately the dental schools, both in the past and present, have not discovered the functional link between the teeth and the craniosacral system. There is a delicate balance between the meshing of the teeth and stability of the twenty-eight skull bones. Not only do the teeth rebalance the cranium but also maintains balance of the muscles, ligaments, cervical vertebrae and pelvis. The functional link that ties the entire system is a membrane system, the dural tube, which surrounds the brain, passes out the base of the skull, attaches to the upper three cervical vertebrae, and continues down to the second sacral tubercle. This reciprocal system functions like a slinky and any distortion from above can effect changes below and vise versa.

Reconstructing a patient's teeth involves a high skill level. Not only must the dentist possess the abilities to prepare the teeth properly, make good temporary crowns, take accurate bite registrations and impressions but equally important is his ability to adjust the biting surfaces of the crowns to balance the skull bones when the teeth come together. This latter task is not taught in the dental schools and is only learned in post-graduate courses. The integrated concept is not taught as a unified package. Osteopaths and chiropractors that specialize in cranial concepts teach the basics of the cranial mechanism. Most dentists are unaware of the existence of this knowledge base. Only through studying both functional dental orthopedics as it relates to the cranium and the cranial mechanism as it relates to dental structures can one begin to recognize how closely knit these two specialties really are. Unfortunately there are very few dental practitioners who have mastered integrating these two fields and capable of providing this type of service.

JM had undergone sinus surgery in an attempt to resolve the facial pain. The ear, nose, and throat specialist made a diagnosis of sinusitis and believed it to be the underlying cause of the patient's problem. Reality soon set in when the post-surgery did not produce the anticipated results. The cause of the chronic facial pain was the inaccurate contact made by the posterior crowns. Improper contact resulted in jamming sutures between skull bones as well as tension placed on the dural membranes within the skull. Treatment involved manually manipulating the skull and judiciously adjusting the bite. The process took four months to complete. The facial pain of twenty-two years resolved.

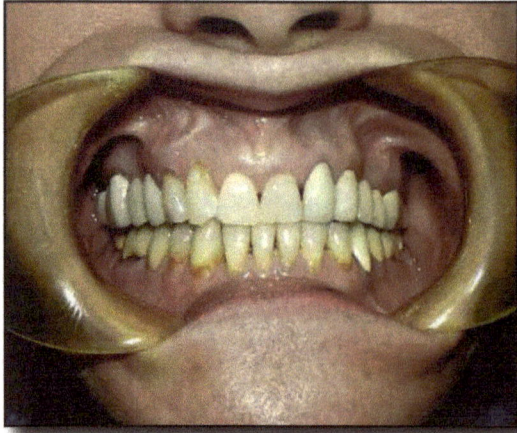

Figure 1

The posterior crowns had biting interferences, which caused jamming of cranial sutures, and placed strain patterns within the patient's skull.

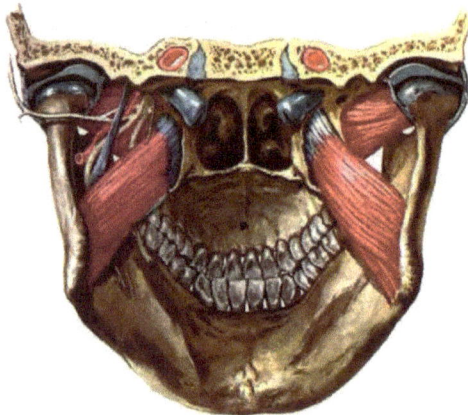

ideal occlusion

Figure 2

An ideal occlusion or balanced bite provides even pressure to the skull bones and balances the muscles and ligaments. The upper teeth are set in the maxilla, which represents the anterior two thirds of the cranial base. If the upper component is distorted (crooked teeth, one side higher than the other) then the forces generated by the teeth will distort the skull. In addition, bite interferences often trigger off muscle spasm, which in turn can jam sutures and distort cranial bone alignment. One of the principal functions of a balanced bite is to serve as a self-correcting mechanism for rebalancing the skull. This rebalancing occurs every time one swallows which is two to three times per minute.

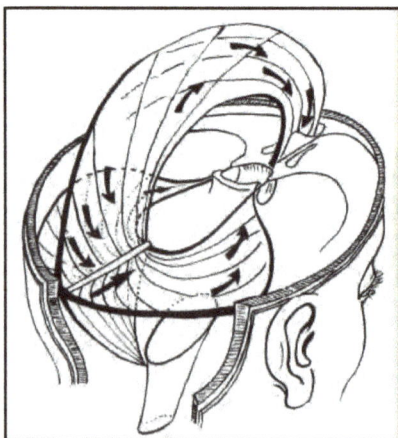

Figure 3 - Referred Pain Patterns

"... tugging on the venous sinuses, damaging the tentorium, or stretching the dura at the base of the brain can all cause intense pain that is recognized as headache. ...almost any type ... of stretching stimulus to the blood vessels of the dura can cause headache."

"Stimulation of pain receptors in the intracranial vault above the tentorium, including the upper tentorium surface itself, initiates impulses in the fifth nerve and therefore causes referred headache to the front half of the head in the area supplied by the fifth cranial nerve."

"..., pain impulses from beneath the tentorium enter the CNS mainly through the second cervical nerve, which also supplies the scalp behind the ear. Therefore, subtentorial pain stimuli cause 'occipital headache' referred to the posterior part of the head."

Guyton, Arthur C., M.D.: Textbook of Medical Physiology. 6th Edition. W.B. Saunders,1981, p.622.

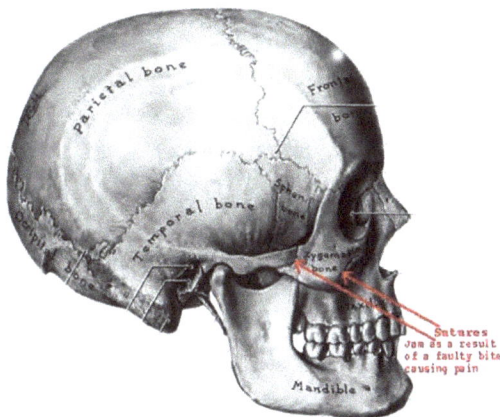

Figure 4 - Cranial Influences

There are twenty-two cranial bones (excluding the six ear ossicles) which function as a synchronized unit. A distortion to one affects the entire unit. The cranial dura is part of the dural tube which extends through the foramen magnum, attaches to the upper three cervical vertebrae and continues down to the second sacral tubercle where it is anchored. Subluxations or fixations anywhere along its path will affect cranial motion. In addition, there are 136 muscles in the head and neck area. Muscle tension or spasm will influence cranial motion. Dental malocclusions in the form of hyper occlusion, deep overbite, crossbite (anterior or posterior), a narrow maxillary arch, faulty crowns or high cant of the maxillae on one side will all have influences on cranial motion.

Twenty Years of Lower Back Pain and Ten Years Right Thigh Pain Resolved

Nate Ostrofsky, who was 87 years young in 2014, presented with a history of 20 years of lower back pain and 10 years of right thigh pain. The patient had a medical history of a left hip replacement and proposed surgical replacement of his right knee. He was referred to our office for evaluation and treatment.

A comprehensive examination revealed cranial bone distortions overlaid by a 15 year old ill-fitting full upper and lower dentures. Initial treatment involved adjusting the cranium to re-establish structural balance with an immediate soft reline of the upper denture to hold the corrected skull alignment. The lower full denture was also relined with a soft material to improve the fit, retention and increase of the vertical height of the dentures. Immediately following the denture relines, the patient stated that his 10 years of right thigh pain totally disappeared. The patient returned two days later to reline the lower denture to further increase the vertical height. Immediately following this procedure, the patient stated that his 20 years of lower back pain improved by 90 percent. Before and after infrared thermal images were taken to objectively document any changes. The post treatment image exhibited a smaller area of pain and a temperature drop of 3.31^0 F. The temperature drop reflects a vasomotor response of the autonomic nervous system. Any temperature reduction greater than 3 degrees is indicative of reduced inflammation.

Loss of vertical height from a worn denture directly causes compression of the spine. Since the temporal bones and the pelvic bones work in unison, a distortion of either of the right or left temporal bone will directly affect the sacroiliac joint. The patient was also seriously contemplating having his right knee surgically replaced. My clinical experience has shown that once the sacroiliac joint is reset to "factory default" the knee issues resolve.

Chapter Five: Dental Complex

Because of a lack of knowledge and an uniformed medical community patients undergo surgical procedures, which in a high percentage of cases could be resolved noninvasively.

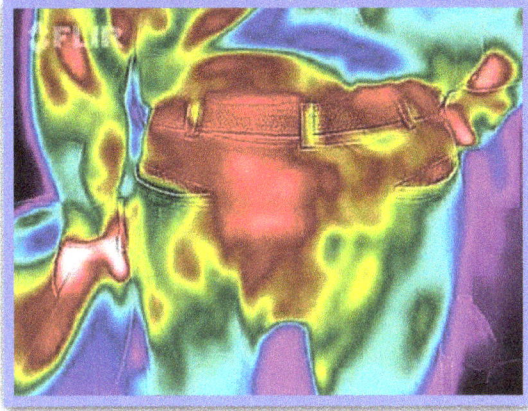

Pre-Treatment Infrared image: The red area depicts the region (sacroiliac) of pain the patient had experienced for the past 20 years.

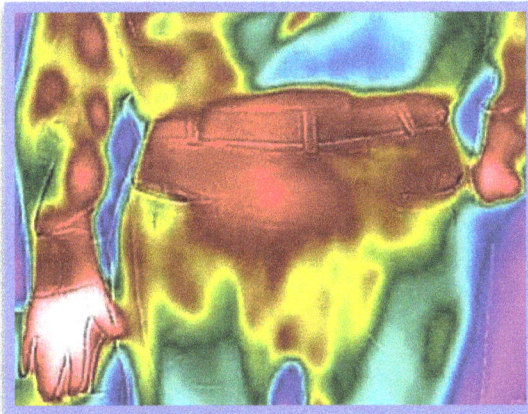

Post-Treatment Infrared image: the red region, which depicts the area of pain, decreased in size. Also the temperature dropped from 70^0 F to 66.69^0 F. The 3.31^0 F drop in temperature occurred immediately following the increase in the vertical height of the lower denture. Changing structural alignment of the cranium and denture directly causes a vasomotor response, that is, the blood vessels relax allowing the stagnated toxins and waste products to get flushed away. With time the patient's symptoms will reduce further.

Atypical Facial Pain/Dental Connection

Patient was referred to our office by her medical doctor for treatment of constant left-side facial and tooth pain. This problem had defied conventional dental treatment for the previous 2 1/2 years. The patient presented with the following:

Chapter Five: Dental Complex

Chief Complaints:

• Left side facial pain and upper left pain in a tooth for 2.5 years.

• Pain in a tooth on the upper right side.

• Anxiety, depression and fatigue.

• Clicking jaw.

• Uneven bite.

• Neck pain.

• **Past Dental History.**

• Upper left first molar:

• First root canal (upper left first molar): Treatment unsuccessful; much pain following treatment.

• Apicoectomy May 1999: Treatment performed by an endodontist (surgical procedure which cuts the tip of the roots off in an attempt to remove area of infection). Treatment was unsuccessful. Constant pain still present.

• Extraction September 1999: Oral surgeon removed failed root canal tooth.

• Second root canal (upper left second molar performed). Pain level not affected.

• Orthodontist and oral surgeon were consulted regarding the TMJ problem. Both concluded that no definitive problem could be seen.

Clinical Findings:

1. Cranial distortions which impacted jaw function.

2. Focus of infection in extraction site: *Staphylococcus, Streptococcus,* osteomylitis (inflammation in jaw bone).

3. Two homeopathic remedies tested positive to resolve infecting agents.

Treatment:

1. Cranial manipulation to correct distortions.

2. Neuro occlusal adjustment to remove bite interferences.

3. Biofrequencies to treat infection in bone.

4. Injected homeopathic remedies into extraction site.

Progress:

Six months of conservative treatment resulted in a 100% reduction in pain.

True biological dentistry focuses on removing the underlying causes of the patient's problem. Each patient must be evaluated to diagnose the specific factors responsible for the symptoms. Each patient must be tested for specific nutrients and dosages to have an effective result. Successful treatment depends on customized care rather than standard protocol that is dished out to all patients presenting with similar symptoms.

X-RAYS
Pre-extraction

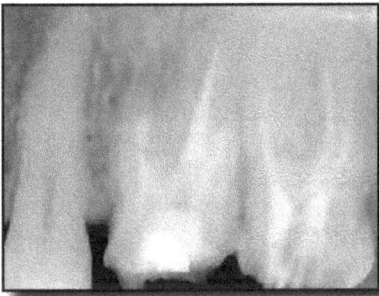

Upper left first molar following root canal and apicoectomy treatment. Conventional treatment was unsuccessful and the patient still experienced constant facial and tooth pain. Mechanically "cleansing" the main canals in a tooth does not resolve the presence of bacterial infection in the dentin tubules. These tiny tubules are 4 microns in diameter and the bacteria are 1 micron. The underlying infections produces toxins which spill out into the periodontal ligament space surrounding the root. This area is highly innervated with nerves which are directly affected by the toxins. The resultant symptom is constant pain.

The upper left first molar was extracted however the pain was still unrelenting. Conventional diagnostic procedures failed to uncover the underlying cause of the patients chronic pain. The bacterial infection migrated into the surrounding bone. The extraction technique did not include a thorough removal of the infected bone that lined the socket. The site "healed" with a residual bacterial infection and perpetuated the constant facial pain even though the tooth was removed.

Post-extraction

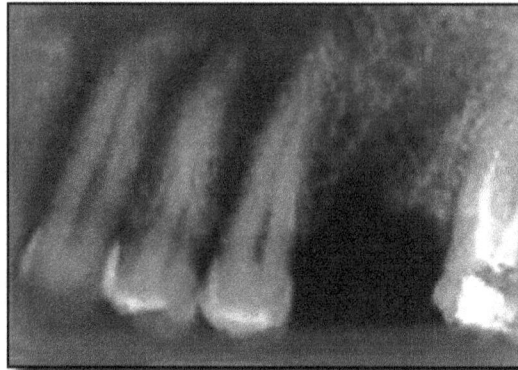

Successful treatment involved injecting specific homeopathic remedies into the bone of the extraction site and the use of biofrequencies to destroy any residual infection not covered by the injections. Mercury removal and nutrients to boost the immune system were adjunctive aides that helped reduce the facial pain by 100%.

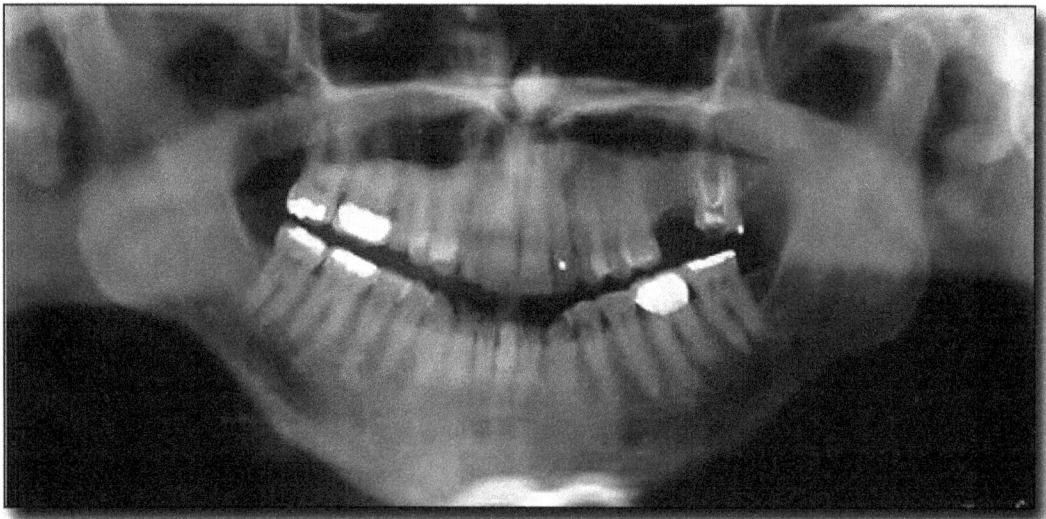

Dental/Menstrual Migraines Connection

When a patient presents with headaches as their chief complaint, they pose a major challenge to the treating practitioner. There are more than 150 different causes for headaches. Different headaches have their own set of symptoms, happen for unique reasons, and need different treatment. The key to unraveling the headache mystery is defining the underlying cause(s).

Heather K. was referred to my office because she had severe migraine headaches. Her migraine headaches were triggered off by her menstrual cycle. Typically Heather would endure severe pain for three days followed by severe fatigue for two weeks. Literally every month Heather was wasted for two weeks.

Typically headaches are caused by illness, stress, and environmental factors. Illness such as an infection, flu, or fever. They are also common with conditions like sinusitis (inflammation of the sinuses), a throat infection, abscessed tooth or an ear infection. In some cases, the headaches may be the result of a concussion or a tumor. Stress: Emotional, chemical, and structural stressors are three factors that distress the adrenal and thyroid glands. Emotional issues along with chemical imbalances, use of alcohol, low blood sugar, sleep disorders, and taking too much medication can also cause headaches. Other stressors include eyestrain and neck or back strain due to subluxations (misalignment of spinal vertebrae) of the spine, pelvis and sacrum.

Environmental factors including secondhand tobacco smoke, strong smells from household chemicals or perfumes, allergens, and certain foods (chocolate, dairy, wines specially those high in tyramine), heavy metals, EMFs (electromagnetic frequencies), too much use of cell phones, artificial sweeteners like Aspartame all have the potential of triggering headaches. Stress, pollution, noise, lighting, and weather changes are other possible triggers.

Heather had a medical history of a chronically infected tooth of two years duration. Also of importance was the fact that the start of her menstrual cycle triggered her migraines. Diagnostically, Heather had an abscessed tooth whose toxins and pathogens were being trapped by her thyroid, which is part of the immune system. Such stressors can create a hypothyroid condition, which also has the potential of elevating the estrogen levels and trigger migraine headaches. In addition, Heather had mercury toxicity, chemical issues, and infection issues.

Treatment focused on removing the infected tooth, placement of ozone into the extraction site to disinfect the bone, and nutrients to detox the chemicals and support her thyroid function. Within three months Heather had a dramatic reduction in her migraines. Presently Heather only gets a migraine that lasts for one day and does not experience any lethargy.

The dental component is a key part of many medical illnesses. Unfortunately, not many health care practitioners have the diagnostic skills to connect the dots and resolve longstanding patient complaints.

Nine Month Follow-Up

Heather K.'s migraines were triggered by her menstrual cycle. Of interest was the fact that three months of initial nutritional therapy along with extraction of an infected molar of two years duration reduced her migraines dramatically. However, Heather still had some minor episodes. The underlying issues was estrogen dominance. Heather's estrogen level was too high. She was placed on an all natural supplement, calcium D-glucarate, which reduced her estrogen level and totally eliminated her migraine headaches. The key was defining the underlying cause.

Drug therapy designed to treat only the symptom of pain over the long run would only worsen the patient. Remember taking NSAIDs (non steroidal anti-inflammatory drugs) over the long run will damage your kidneys and liver. If you play you will pay.

Reversing Congestive Heart Failure the Old Fashioned Way! Nutrition/Dental Infections/Heart Failure Connection

Every patient is a chemical individual and must be examined to determined the source (infections in the jaw bone, nutritional deficiencies, damaged heart muscle, nerve degeneration, heavy metal toxicity, etc.) of their congestive heart failure. It is also imperative that each patient be tested for supplements that will neutralize their specific problem. Using a standard protocol for all CHF patients is not realistic and greatly reduces ones chances for success.

The following case study is being presented to demonstrate that in certain situations congestive heart failure can be reversed. This study is not intended to suggest that all congestive heart patients can be treated with the same protocol. This case study is being presented in the hope that interest will be stimulated among physicians and patients to explore an integrated approach to this most serious malady that is plaguing our population.

Case Study: 73-Year-Old Caucasian Male Diagnosed with Congestive Heart Failure.

History of Present Illness: The patient was admitted 08/18/99 to the Lourdes Hospital intensive care unit with severe fatigue, hallucinations, confusion, nausea and vomiting. He was found to be in severe bi-ventricular heart failure and was treated initially with intravenous inotropic support in the form of Dobutamine and given intravenous diuretics. He was seen by a local cardiologist. The patient had brief runs of non-sustained ventricular tachycardia, as well as episodes of supraventricular tachycardia which, upon review, appeared to be paroxysmal atrial tachycardia, atrial flutter and possibly one episode of atrial fibrillation. Echocardiogram showed severe mitral insufficiency and severe left ventricular dysfunction. The estimated ejection fraction was approximately 15 to 20%. There was some suggestion of left ventricular thrombi for which the patient was started on Heparin and then Coumadin.

The patient, Walter Kruse, was in hospice waiting to die. Because of Walter's age, a heart transplant was not available. Medical testing performed by Kennedy Memorial Hospitals revealed the following findings:
(7/13/99):

- No blocked coronary arteries.

- Abnormal left ventricular contractility of a dilated left ventricle with severe reduction in the overall left ventricular systolic function. The ejection fraction estimated at 15-20%.

- There is mild mitral valve regurgitation.

- Severe pulmonary hypertension is present.

- Within three months after the first evaluation the patient's heart deteriorated. The mild mitral valve regurgitation progressed to severe.

University of Pennsylvania Health System
Echocardiography Report 10/26/99:

- Moderate biatrial enlargement. Moderate right and left ventricular enlargement.

- Evidence of severe cardiomyopathy involving the left ventricle.

- Mitral valve is structurally normal although there is severe regurgitation.

- Moderate tricuspid valve regurgitation.

- Severe pulmonary hypertension.

- Aortic valve is sclerotic without stenosis. There is trace regurgitation.

During the interim period between October 26, 1999 and June 16, 2000, Walter Kruse was placed on a custom nutritional supplement program specifically designed to support repair of heart tissue strengthen the mitral value and right ventricle. Because of the severity of the patient's condition, Walter was taking 80 vitamins per day. Within approximately 7 months the following documented changes were independently recorded by a medical facility.

Shore Memorial Hospital
Cardiac Diagnostics 6/16/00

• Tricuspid valve - Within normal limits.

• Mitral valve - Within normal limits.

• Left ventricle - Estimated ejection fraction 40-50%.

• Right ventricle - Normal in size and systolic function.

• Aortic valve - Within normal limits.

• Right and left atria - Mildly dilated.

Congestive heart failure (CHF) is a common condition within our population. CHF affects more than 4.5 million people in the USA, with nearly half a million new cases being diagnosed each year. It is also estimated that nearly 20 million people have unsuspected heart failure and are likely to develop symptoms in the next 1-5 years. The many symptoms of CHF result from the inability of the heart to pump adequate amounts of blood to the various parts of the body (e.g., brain, arms, legs, organs, tissues) and the fluid back-up that results within the organs. A decreased blood supply to the brain results in dizziness, and the legs will often become swollen with fluid. When the blood pressure drops because of a weakened heart muscle, the kidneys cannot properly remove the waste products from the blood. The direct result is kidney failure, which causes the body to build up toxic waste and eventually causes the death of the patient.

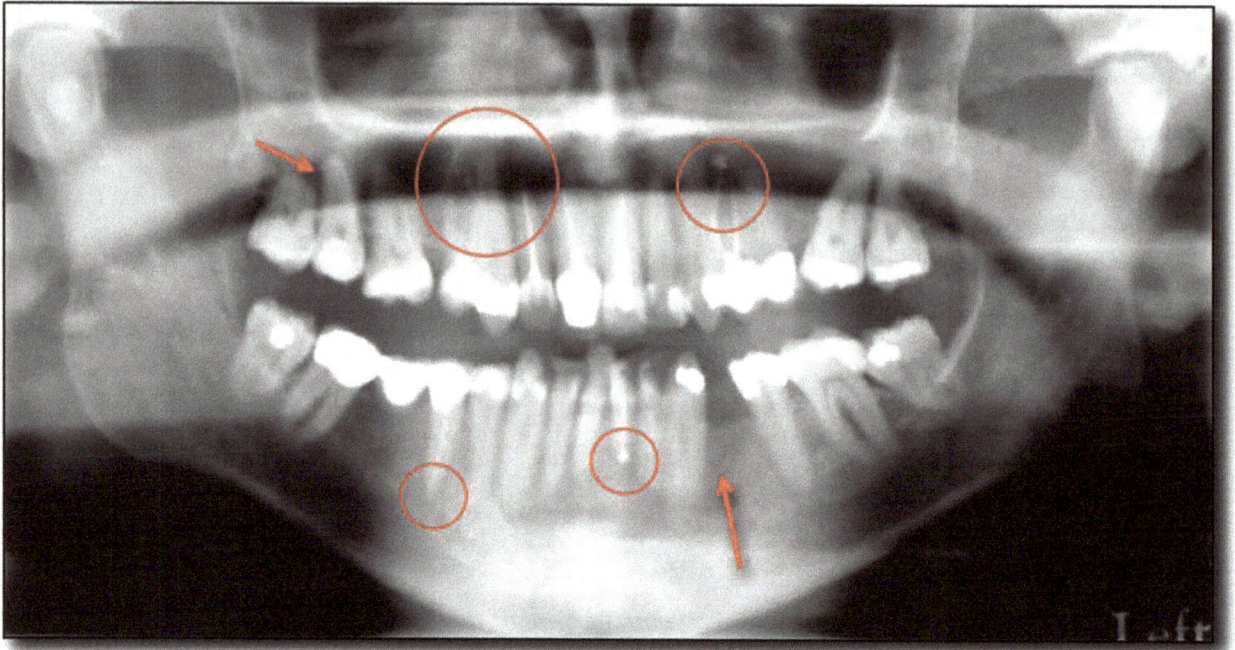

Walter Kruse's Panoramic radiograph depicts a super toxic waste dump. All the fancy dentistry which includes root canals, gold crowns, apicoectomy (surgical procedure to fill the end of the root tip with a mercury filling), mercury fillings contribute to create toxins (mercury, thioethers, mercaptan, and hydrogen sulfide from the root canal teeth, galvanic or electrical currents from the dissimilar metals in the mouth) which will ultimately drain into the thyroid. Toxicity in the thyroid causes hypothyroidism which will weaken the heart.

Traditional medicine treats CHF with medications (Diuretics, ACE inhibitors, Angiotensin-2 blockers, Carvedilol and Digitalis. Other drugs that may be used in the treatment of CHF include spironolactone (which has been shown to preserve potassium and reduce the deterioration of CHF), "blood thinners" (that reduce the risk of blood clots), anti-arrhythmic agents (to treat dangerous irregular heart beats), and blood pressure medications (when ACE inhibitors are unable to control the high blood pressure) are contraindicated. By integrating medications when appropriately indicated with specific nutrients to feed the heart muscles, the patient has a much better chance of reversing the cardiac damage. Employing an orthodox approach of only drugs, greatly reduces the patient's chances of repairing their heart. It must be clearly understood that NOT All patients can be reversed. Sometimes the damage is too extensive and the overall state of health is very poor which precludes any success. Each patient must be evaluated on their own merits and their own findings will then dictate which treatment protocols should be used.

Traditional allopathic medicine provides the same protocol for all patients with the same symptoms. This treatment approach often times does not address the patient's problems.

For six years, Walter Kruse lived a full and productive life. He was healthier after treatment than before his congestive heart episode. The documentation showed that in this patient the mitral valve and right ventricle did heal. Walter is living testimony that there is a better way. Unfortunately, at the six year mark, his cardiologist changed his medication from digitoxin to Coreg. Coreg has a major adverse side effect, throwing blood clots. His physician prescribed a dose four times greater than what he should have had, and he died.

Death by Medicine.

By Gary Null, PhD; Carolyn Dean MD, ND; Martin Feldman, MD; Debora Rasio, MD; and Dorothy Smith, PhD.

"Something is wrong when regulatory agencies pretend that vitamins are dangerous, yet ignore published statistics showing that government-sanctioned medicine is the real hazard."

Full article can be viewed at: **www.webdc.com/pdfs/deathbymedicine.pdf**

Stage IV Dental Cancer Connection

When Roland was diagnosed with stage IV throat cancer and told his endocrinologist he was going the alternative route, the doctor told him it was a farce and he was wasting his time and money. Roland was referred to my office for evaluation and treatment of infected root canal teeth.

Roland's hospital report documented stage IV throat cancer with bilateral swollen cervical lymph nodes.

DX: Three infected teeth were present: lower left second bicuspid and second molar and maxillary left second molar.

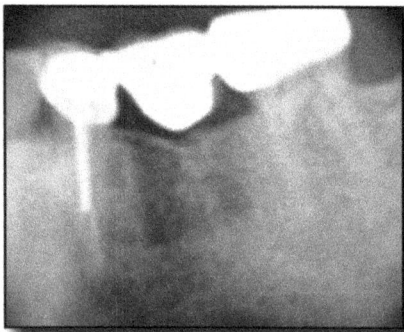

The same pathogens (*Streptococcus viridans* and *Tuberculinum*) present in the three teeth were also present in the swollen cervical lymph nodes and throat cancer.

Tx: Extraction of the three infected teeth plus irrigation with ozone, colloidal silver, and homeopathic remedies in the extraction site; biofrequencies, raw juices, food-based supplements and Insulin Potentiation Therapy totally resolved the cancer in three weeks.

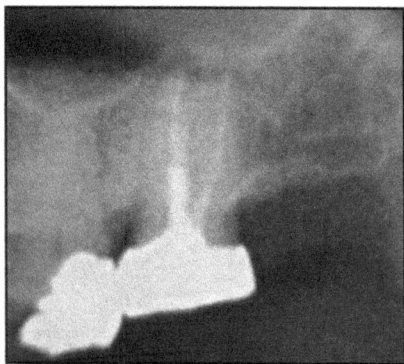

When Roland confronted his endocrinologist at the hospital he asked him that he wanted to speak to the doctor's other cancer patients and tell them what alternative treatments were available, the doctor would not speak with him. So much for academic honesty and the War on Cancer. Roland has been cancer free since 2009.

Chapter Five: Dental Complex

Dentistry is the only profession that embalms an organ and keeps it in the body. This is insanity. A dead organ in the body creates a constant source of inflammation derived from the putrefaction of dead tissue. In addition, one of the toxic chemicals produced from decaying protein is thioethers, which is a derivative of mustard gas. All toxins from the mouth drain via the lymphatic system into the thyroid, thymus and rest of the body. This toxic overload suppresses the immune system.

The Toxic Element Research Foundation (TERF), using state of the art DNA testing technology, identified multiple pathological bacteria found within root canal teeth, the bone adjacent to the teeth, and even more in extraction sites where healing has not taken place. This non–healing occurs in greater than 99 percent of wisdom tooth extraction sites. Additionally, large defects of non-healing are often found upon surgical exploration into the bone – about the size of the original wisdom tooth. Other sites leave what are called "cavitations" as well.

In the 1950s, Dr. Josef Issels of Germany found that in his 40 years of treating "terminal" cancer patients, 97 percent of his cancer patients had root canals. He would not initiate his successful treatments until all root canals had been removed.

Dr. Weston Price — head of research for the American Dental Association for 14 years in the 1920s and 30s — published the results of 1000 extracted teeth in which canal sterilization was done in the dental research laboratory. Researchers in the laboratory used not just the routine sterilizing chemicals but extremely potent sterilizing agents (more toxic than could possibly be used in the mouth) and in a highly controlled sterile environment. Their microbiology specialists found that 97 percent were cultured to find re–contamination within 48 hours. In other words, they were still infected.

The toxicity of root canals was disclosed by Mayo's Clinic and Dr. Weston Price jointly back in about 1910. Close to a century ago. Price's textbook on root canals, published in 1922, upset the dental associations at that time and still does today. The American Dental Association (ADA), denies his findings and claims that they have proven root canals to be safe; however, no published data from the ADA is available to confirm this statement. Statements, but no actual research.

Lunacy of "Modern" Dentistry: Chronic Dental Pain Pathogen Connection

Dawn M. had chronic pain in her lower right canine tooth for four years. She had a root canal treatment done twice. The pain still persisted. Then the geniuses talked her into having a gamma knife procedure performed. That didn't work either. The pain still persisted. Then another genius talked her into having cranial surgery to try to relieve the "pressure" off the trigeminal nerve. Again another failure, and the pain still persisted.

Using the Quantum Testing Technique, two pathogens showed up around the apex or tip of the lower right canine root: herpes simplex I and herpes zoster (shingles). Biofrequency therapy was applied for two weeks, and the pain was reduced by fifty percent. The pain still remained at the reduced level. My recommendation was to remove the offending root canal tooth. Immediately following the extraction and after the periodontal ligaments were meticulously curetted out, ozone was injected into the extraction site followed by colloidal silver and Sanum homeopathic remedies.

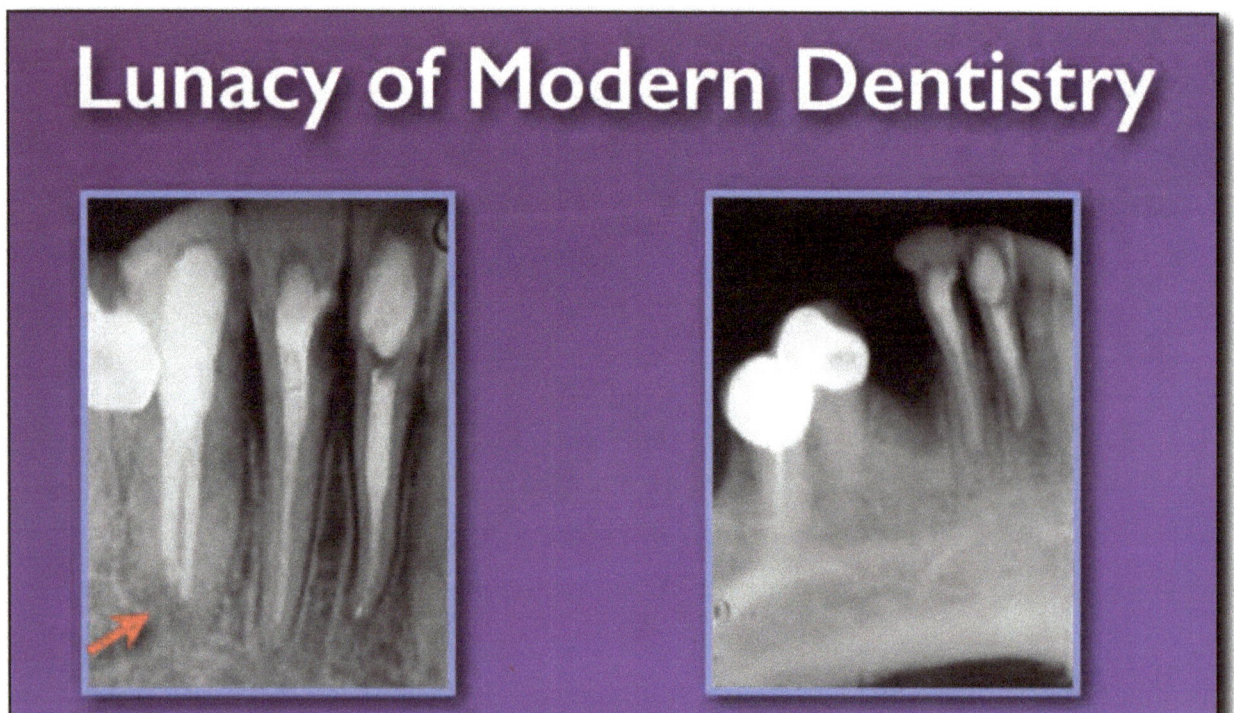

Chapter Five: Dental Complex

The pain totally resolved. All the sophisticated gold standard testing could not make an accurate diagnosis. Only energy testing technique can get to the core issue quickly, accurately, and noninvasively. Traditional testing is obsolete because it does not pick up what is trapped in the embalmed tooth and surrounding bone and soft tissues.

Fifteen Years of Vertigo Caused by a Root Canal Treated Tooth

Duncan A. suffered sever vertigo for fifteen years. He had to sleep with two pillows to counteract the spinning sensation. He was also unable to fly. Medical examination at Johns Hopkins University, Hershey Medical Center, and treatment with numerous neurologists failed to diagnose Duncan's underlying cause.

Duncan came in for an extended examination. A major red flag went up when Duncan mentioned he had a lower left second molar that was treated with root canal therapy. When the tooth was tested by means of an energetic technique it showed the presence of infection with cytomegalovirus. Also this same virus was present in his left inner ear, which was the same side Duncan experienced his vertigo. Treatment involved specific nutrients and home treatment with his own Bio-frequency device (Rife Functional Generator). Two months into treatment his left ear popped open and his vertigo vanished. Duncan has been free of all his vertigo symptoms for the past several years.

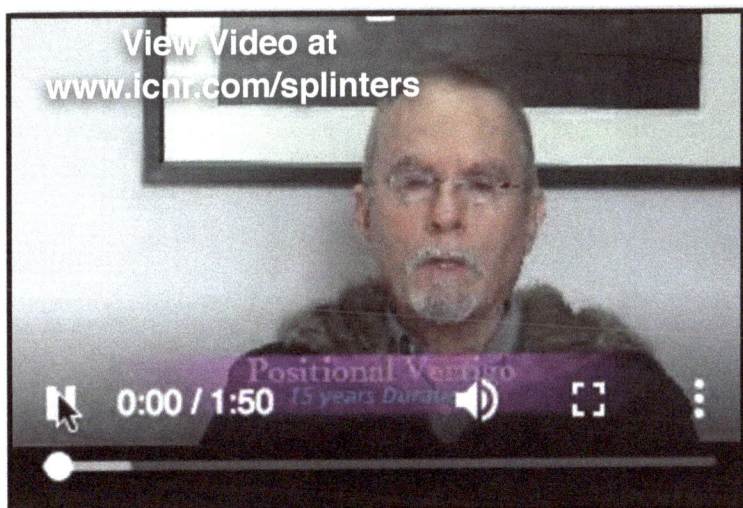

Chapter Five: Dental Complex

There is much controversy surrounding the concept of root canal therapy; however, after reading the scientific literature and reviewing the cases presented in this book, one does not have to be a rocket scientist to realize that a dead organ has the potential for causing severe health issues.

Mercury Basal Cell Cancer Connection

A retired dentist presented with basal cell carcinoma on the right side of her nose. The cancerous lesion was present for one year. During that period Andrea B. did wheatgrass juice, acupuncture, vitamins and herbs with no results. The focus of this book is on defining the core problem, which is not being done by most practitioners. Again using Quantum Testing Technique, it revealed that mercury was in the cancerous lesion. You can do all the "right" therapies but if they do not address the causative factor(s), the "disease" will not go away. In essence, cancer is NOT a disease. It is a breakdown of the immune system and corruption of the cell membranes preventing adequate levels of oxygen to pass into the cell.

Mercury is the second most toxic substance on this planet second only to plutonium. Mercury gives off between thirteen and 20 different frequencies that disrupt the physiology of the cell and corrupts the cell membrane. Mercury has an affinity for tubulin, the fatty insulation that surrounds nerve fibers. Heavy metals like mercury corrupt the cell membranes specially disrupting the omega-6 component within the unsaturated part of the cell. It is the omega-6 component that acts as a magnet pulling in the oxygen into the cell. When the oxygen level drops by 35%, the cell goes into survival mode. Low oxygen initiates fermentation which converts glucose into lactic acid. Over time the cells transform into cancer cells. The solution is simple. First, remove the "splinter" mercury. Second, repair the cell membrane by supplying organic sulfur in the form of MSM (methyl sulfonyl methane); third, supply organic and cold pressed omega-6 fatty acid to rebuild the cell membrane; and fourth, supply cordyceps to increase the ATP (adenosin triphosphate) in the mitochondria to increase energy production. Giving the body ozone is a great way to turbo charge the cells and destroy chemicals, pathogens and any other toxins. In addition, it is crucial to provide an efficient systemic enzyme to dissolve away the biofilm surrounding the cancer cells, which provide protection from being recognized by the body's own immune system. Furthermore the body produces fibrin in response to chronic inflammation. The excess fibrin hampers microcirculation and also makes the cell membrane less permeable.

The patient went through three major detox phases as a means of expelling the mercury and other toxins. At the end of one year and three months the cancer healed. Isn't that amazing? When you remove the "splinters," the body goes back to "factory default." This paradigm applies to all medical issues, autoimmune disease, fibromyalgia, Crohn's disease, arthritis, AIDS, dementia, and so forth. The problem in our sick care system is that physicians are not trained to uncover the real cause. They are only trained to treat the symptoms.

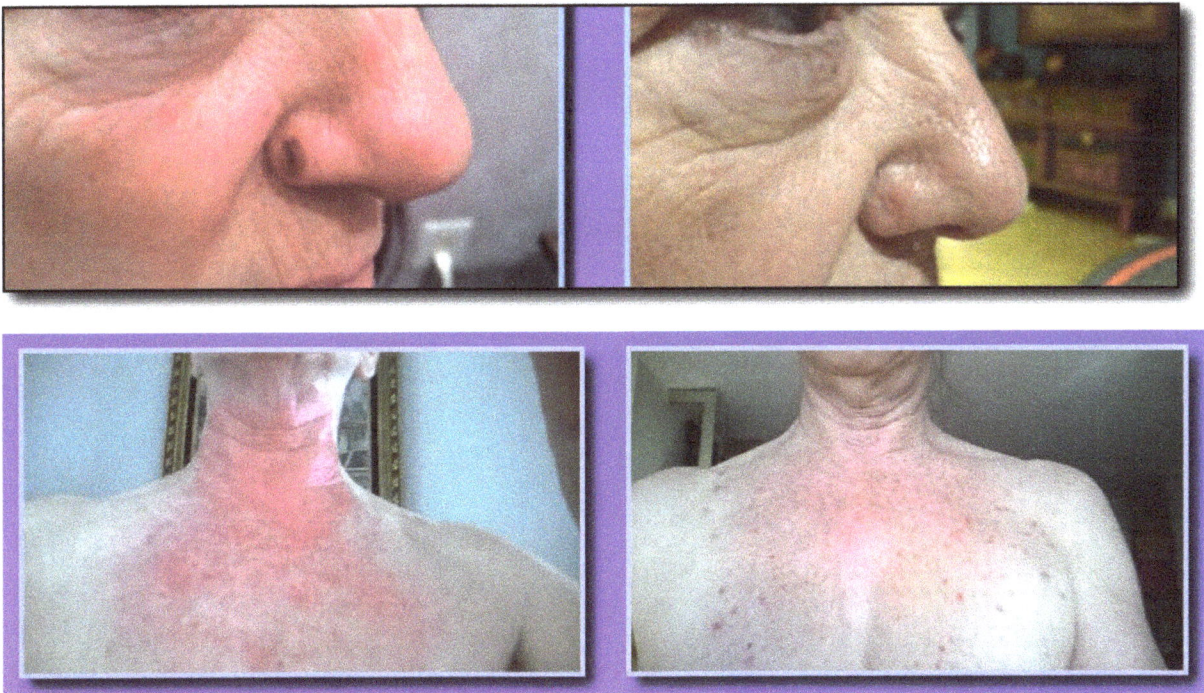

Typical detox reactions involve rashes, flu-like symptoms, headaches, achy joints, fever, diarrhea, hemorrhoids, bad breath, acne, fatigue, constipation, and frequent urination. When food-based nutrients are taken, the body purges the toxins.

Lung Cancer Root Canal Connection

Carol K. developed right lung cancer. Neanderthal conventional treatment cut off the tip of her right lung where the cancer was present. The patient refused chemo or any other traditional treatment. Six months later the cancer appeared in the left lung. The reason is simple. The underlying cause was not removed. Again the patient refused any surgical intervention. Carol was then referred to my office by her chiropractor.

As part of the comprehensive examination, the patient was requested to bring in her pathology slides of the cancerous tissues. Using Quantum Testing Technique, it was discovered that there were three "splinters" in Carol's cancerous tissues: a pesticide, cytomegalovirus, and mercury. A nutrition program was formulated to remove the three "splinters," detox the liver and clean up her body. In six months Carols' cancer disappeared. The solution was hidden in plain view but conventional medicine cannot see it.

ROOT CANAL/ LUNG CANCER

Pathology slides were tested energetically

CMV

Quantum Testing Dx: CMV, Hg, and a pesticide in the cancerous tissue!

The root canal tooth was infected with the cytomegalovirus, the same virus that was in the cancerous tissue. Do you think there is a connection? The tooth was extracted, ozonated, and cleansed with colloidal silver and homeopathic remedies.

Nobel Prize Winner, Otto Warburg, M.D., P.h.D. Discovers The Real Cause of Cancer

In 1931, Otto Warburg, M.D., P.h.D. won a Nobel Prize in Physiology for his discovery for the cause of cancer. He stated, "the prime cause of cancer is the replacement of the respiration of oxygen in normal body cells by a fermentation of sugar." Dr. Warburg uncovered part of the equation of cancer. What he did not figure out was the reason for the low oxygen levels. The initiating factor is adulterated omega-6 fatty acids. The adulterated oils corrupt the cell membrane, which interferes with its ability to transport the oxygen across the cell membrane into the cell. When oxygen drops by thirty-five percent over time, the cell shifts into survival mode and reverts to fermentation to break down the glucose (sugar). Over time cells deprived of sufficient oxygen mutate and cause cancer.

Besides detoxing the body and taking anti-oxidant supplements, one has to supply the body with unadulterated organic, cold pressed omega-6 fatty acids (safflower oil, sunflower oil, black currant seed oil, borage oil, pumpkin seed oil, and walnut oil) to repair the cell membranes. It is the omega-6 fatty acids which act as the magnet pulling in the oxygen. Unfortunately, most if not all processed foods and restaurants use adulterated oil to prepare their food. The only answer is to supplement.

The medical establishment has the physicians and public snowed when it comes to the topic of cancer. The oncologists truly believe that there are numerous types of cancer. Dr. Warburg proved that there is one one type of cancer and it's caused by an oxygen deficiency.When this abnormality occurs in the ovaries, the cancer takes on the characteristics of the ovarian cells. If it occurs in the breasts, the characteristics of the cancer are similar to breast cells. It just depends on where the process initiates.

The "splinter" theory espoused by this author focuses on defining the causative agents, repair of the cell membranes, detoxification of all the defined pollutants, correcting the body's pH, feeding the system real food, eliminating as many variables as possible, and having the patient change their attitude about themselves and work on erasing the pre-recorded tapes from childhood. Only a comprehensive approach has the best chance of resolving cancer. Remember cancer is NOT a disease; it is an oxygen deficiency coupled with a toxic body environment.

Toxic Root Canal Teeth

Doctor Weston A. Price was on a mission to solve the root canal issue. Two weeks after he performed a root canal on his son, Donald, his son died of endocarditis. Doctor Price extracted the tooth from his son and placed the contaminated dead roots under the skin of two hundred consecutive healthy rabbits. All the rabbits died of endocarditis just like his son.

Dr. Price took one thousand extracted teeth and reamed them out as dentists normally do prior to filling the canals with gutta-percha (filling material used for root canal teeth). Price sterilized the canals with forty different chemicals far too toxic to be used in a live human situation; he wanted to see whether the canals could be permanently sterilized. After forty-eight hours, each tooth was broken apart and cultured for the presence of bacteria. Nine hundred and ninety teeth out of one thousand cultured toxic bacteria just two days after treatment with chemicals designed to make the teeth sterile. Where did these bacteria come from?

The dental complex represents a major potential interference field that can wreak havoc with the entire body. To really appreciate the role the stomatognathic system plays, one must study and integrate osteopathic, chiropractic principles, plus the field of physiology, nutrition, physical therapy, quantum physics, energy medicine, acupuncture, cranial manipulation, homeopathy, meditation, and other natural healing modalities. Because professional schools have a four year window to teach their students the basics, their curriculums cannot accommodate the broad spectrum of information required to have a working knowledge of true healing. Because of this major hurdle, their students graduate with just the basics to conduct a general practice. It takes approximately eight to ten years of being in the field for the doctor to wake up and be able to afford the time to take the necessary post-graduate courses to learn how the human body works on a functional basis. This lack of information is the underlying reason why patients slip through the proverbial cracks in the healthcare system. Until this situation is remedied, our healthcare system will continue to provide incomplete treatments primarily focused on symptomatic relief.

Pelvic Complex

In 1982, I joined a chiropractic study group in Marlton, New Jersey. That was the beginning of my journey to piece the grand puzzle together. One of the chiropractors in the study group invited me to take my first post-graduate chiropractic seminar in the Meadowlands in New Jersey. Lawrence DeMann, D.C., was a well-known Sacro-Occipital Technique (SOT) practitioner who presented the concept of the cranium, temporomandibular joint, and the pelvis. Dr. DeMann gave an in-depth discussion of each of the components and their functional interrelationship. At that time, I did not fully understand the mechanics of what he presented; however, I did walk away with an overall picture of how they had the potential to affect one another. I also realized that Dr. DeMann did not have a comprehensive understanding of how the bite (occlusion) influenced the temporomandibular joint (TMJ), the cranium, and the pelvis. It literally took me 35 years of additional post-graduate seminars and clinical experience to discover how the dental complex related to the rest of the body. Once I mastered the intricacies of how the system worked and successfully applied the principles clinically, miracles began to happen.

In 1988, I attended a seminar given by two applied kinesiologists, Drs. Herb Anderson and Carl Ferrari. They taught me the muscle interlinks that existed between the chewing muscles and the pelvic muscles. The following table shows the specific muscles and their functional interlink.

Chewing Muscles	**Pelvic Muscles**
1. Masseter	Gluteus medius and gluteus minimus
2. Buccinator	Obturator Internus
3. Temporalis	Quadratus lumborum
4. Internal pterygoid	Psoas
5. External pterygoid	Leg Adductors

In terms of functional anatomy, this means if any one of the chewing muscles goes into dysfunction or spasm the contralateral or opposite side muscle interlink will be directly affected. The same holds true from below the body moving upward. If a specific pelvic muscle becomes dysfunctional, its opposite upper interlink partner reacts. For example, if the lower left psoas muscle, which attaches to the intervertebral discs in the lower back, goes into spasm its opposite interlink on the upper right, the internal pterygoid muscle, will react. From a treatment perspective, if your pain is in the low back but its origin is coming from a spasm in the upper internal pterygoid interlink muscle, treatment of the lower back muscle will be ineffective. Clinically, the practitioner would be treating the wagging tail of the dog and not the source. If the therapy you are getting from a practitioner is not working, he or she has not discovered the root cause. The healthcare practitioner must have a working knowledge of these interrelationships in order to solve the problem.

One major factor that eludes many practitioners is the presence of an underactive thyroid. Most blood tests do not reveal this problem. One of the side effects of hypothyroidism is weak muscles and ligaments. If the underactive thyroid is not addressed, no amount of manipulation will stabilize the sacroiliac joint of the pelvic complex. One accurate way of diagnosing an underactive thyroid is to take your armpit temperature for 30 days first thing in the morning before getting out of bed. If your temperature readings are consistently below 97.8^0 F, your thyroid is not working properly. This concept is based on 20 years of arduous research conducted by Dr. Broda Barnes. Unfortunately, the medical establishment has ignored this brilliant work.

Pelvis and Ligaments, Rear View, Female

The red arrow points to the sacroiliac joint.

The pelvis is held together purely by ligaments. From a functional perspective, the innominate or pelvic bones reciprocate with the temporal bones where the temporomandibular joint articulates. Any disturbance in the temporal bones potentially affects the innominate bones. If a patient presents with a loss of vertical support on one side, the sacroiliac joint on the same side becomes misaligned.

Since there are direct muscle interlinks between the chewing muscles and the pelvic muscles, many patients who suffer from sciatic pain really have a dental problem that has not been recognized.

Dental—Sciatic Pain Connection

Patients with relentless sciatic pain have a tremendous burden to bear. Living with any kind of pain is not pleasant, but sciatic pain can be especially disabling. A primary symptom is sciatic neuralgia or pain starting from the buttocks and shooting down the back of the leg and sometimes into different portions of the lower leg. The sciatic nerve runs right through the belly of the piriformis muscle, and if the piriformis muscle contracts from being overused the sciatic nerve now becomes entrapped, producing pain, tingling, and numbness. Sciatic pain can come from many different sources (i.e., a herniated disc, a pronated foot, upper cervical dysfunction); however, one origin is not too well known: that of dental/cranial distortions.

The Sacro-Occipital Technique developed by Major B. DeJarnette, D.C. and Applied Kinesiology developed by George Goodheart, D.C. are two chiropractic concepts that provide a global approach designed to treat the body more comprehensively. The functional connection lies in the dural tube, which connects the cranial dental complex, the spine, and the sacral/pelvic complex. The so-called "slinky" effect clearly describes this system. Two applied kinesiologists, Drs. Herbert Anderson and Carl Ferrari, recognized and demonstrated that there is a direct muscle interlink between the chewing muscles and the gluteus medius, obturator internus, quadratus lumborium, and psoas and leg adductors, which help stabilize the pelvis. Another connecting link stems from the Lovett Brother relationship, which relates specific bone interlinks between the skull and pelvic complex. Distortions from either end will reflect upward or downward, and the structures in between will compensate.

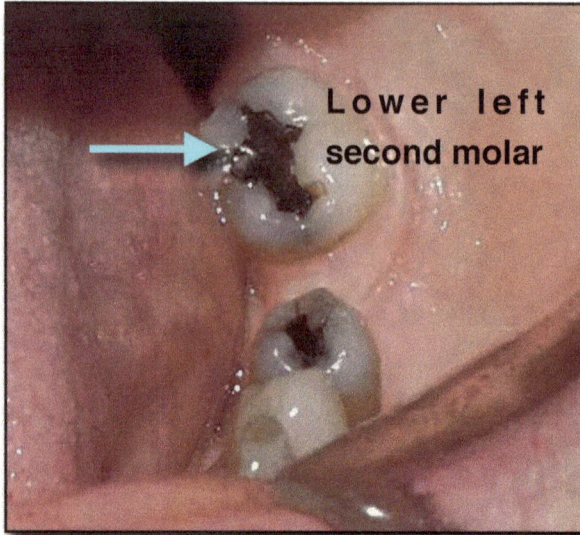

Lower left
second molar

Norma B. suffered with constant sciatic pain for three years. Neurologists, chiropractors, physical therapists and medical doctors could not resolve her pain. Norma's quality of life was non-existent. At her daughter's request, Norma made an appointment to get evaluated. She presented with a primary cranial/dental distortion accompanied by a primary pronation of the feet. Severe scoliosis was also present. When tested, her left piriformis muscle was weak. Interestingly, when her cranium was rebalanced and a "shim" placed on one tooth to support her skull alignment, the left piriformis muscle immediately strengthened. In 90 minutes of treatment, Norma got up from the dental chair and in total disbelief stated that her sciatic pain was totally gone. The key to successful treatment was the fact that the underlying structural imbalances were diagnosed and properly treated.

A "shim" was placed on the lower right second molar to level the cranial bone

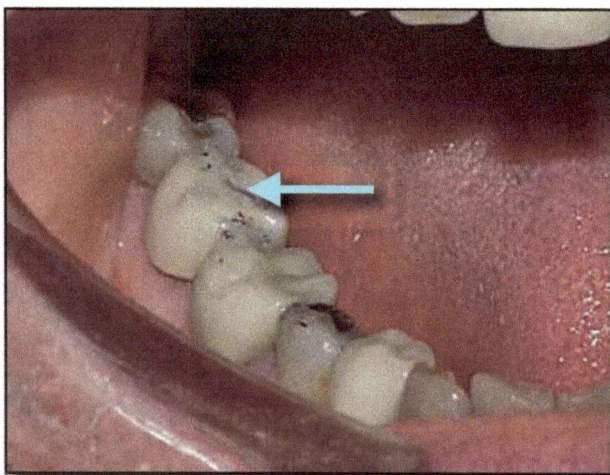

alignment, which eliminated the compression of the sciatic nerve by the piriformis muscle.

A minor occlusal interference was removed from the lower left second molar. This neurological abnormality of the bite was a factor in causing the weakness of the left piriformis muscle.

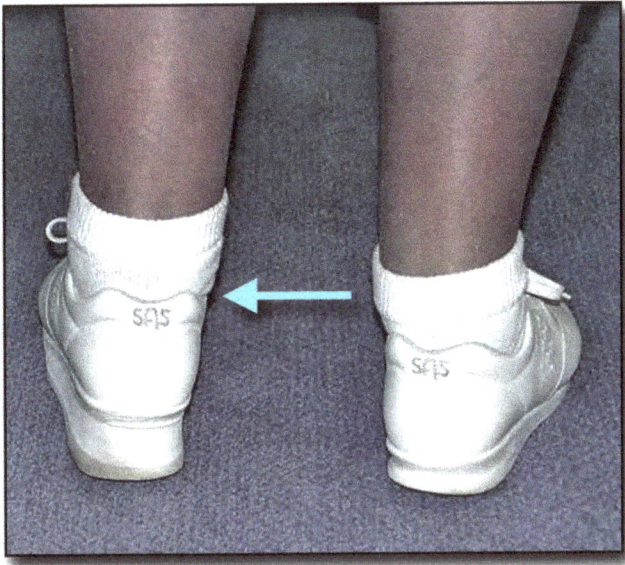

Norma had bilateral pronation (the arch is flat and the ankles cave inward). The pronation of the right foot was worse than that of the left. Norma's therapist placed a 6 mm proprioceptive stimulator in both shoes to correct the structural imbalance.

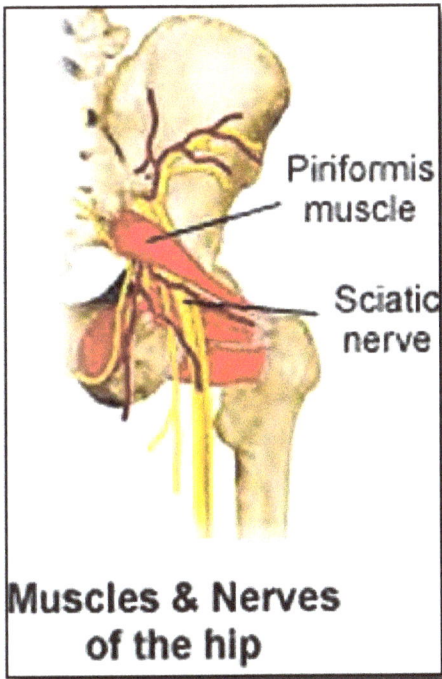

Piriformis muscle

Sciatic nerve

Muscles & Nerves of the hip

The function of the piriformis muscle can be directly affected by a malocclusion and/or mechanical interference in the bite. The piriformis muscle is attached to the sacrum, which is directly influenced by the teeth.

Months of Low Back Pain Resolved with One Cranial Adjustment

Michele Capriotti came to my office after listening to a radio interview by Jonathan Landsman.

Michele had suffered low back pain for months with no resolution from chiropractic, massage, and other body work. A whiplash event set the stage for disrupting her cranial bone alignment, which was not diagnosed by any of the professionals who worked on her.

In just one twenty-minute session, to Michele's amazement I was able to correct her distortions and her low back pain totally disappeared.

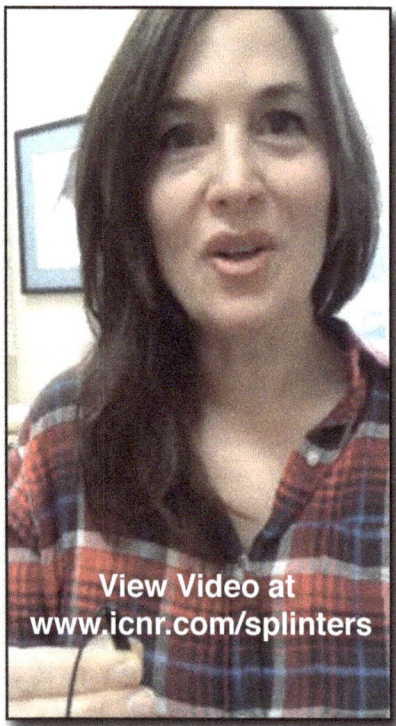

View Video at
www.icnr.com/splinters

Even though cranial manipulation was discovered and implemented as far back as the 1930s, very few practitioners utilize this powerful treatment. It is a sad commentary that noninvasive therapies such as cranial manipulation exist and can alleviate much pain and suffering but they still go unnoticed and unrecognized by the healthcare establishment.

"The doctor of the future will give no medicine, will interest his patient in the care of the human frame, in diet, and in the cause, and prevention of disease."

Thomas A. Edison 1903

Thirty Years of Suffering Scoliosis Dramatically Improved in One Treatment

Dental—Scoliosis Connection

Dino developed scoliosis following orthodontic four bicuspid amputation and retraction procedures. Conventional orthodontic treatment has the great potential for torquing (twisting) the cranial bones and retracting the mandible. This combination of distortions results in scoliosis by twisting the dural membrane, which extends from the cranium to the sacrum. Also, retracting the lower jaw decreases the vertical height of the bite, which in turn causes compression of the spine. Despite chiropractic treatment, physical therapy, exercises, and acupuncture, no positive results were obtained. Dino's temporal bones were severely torqued with little tooth contact on the posterior left side and pronated feet (arches caved inward), which contributes to the ascending distortion up the spine to the temporal bones.

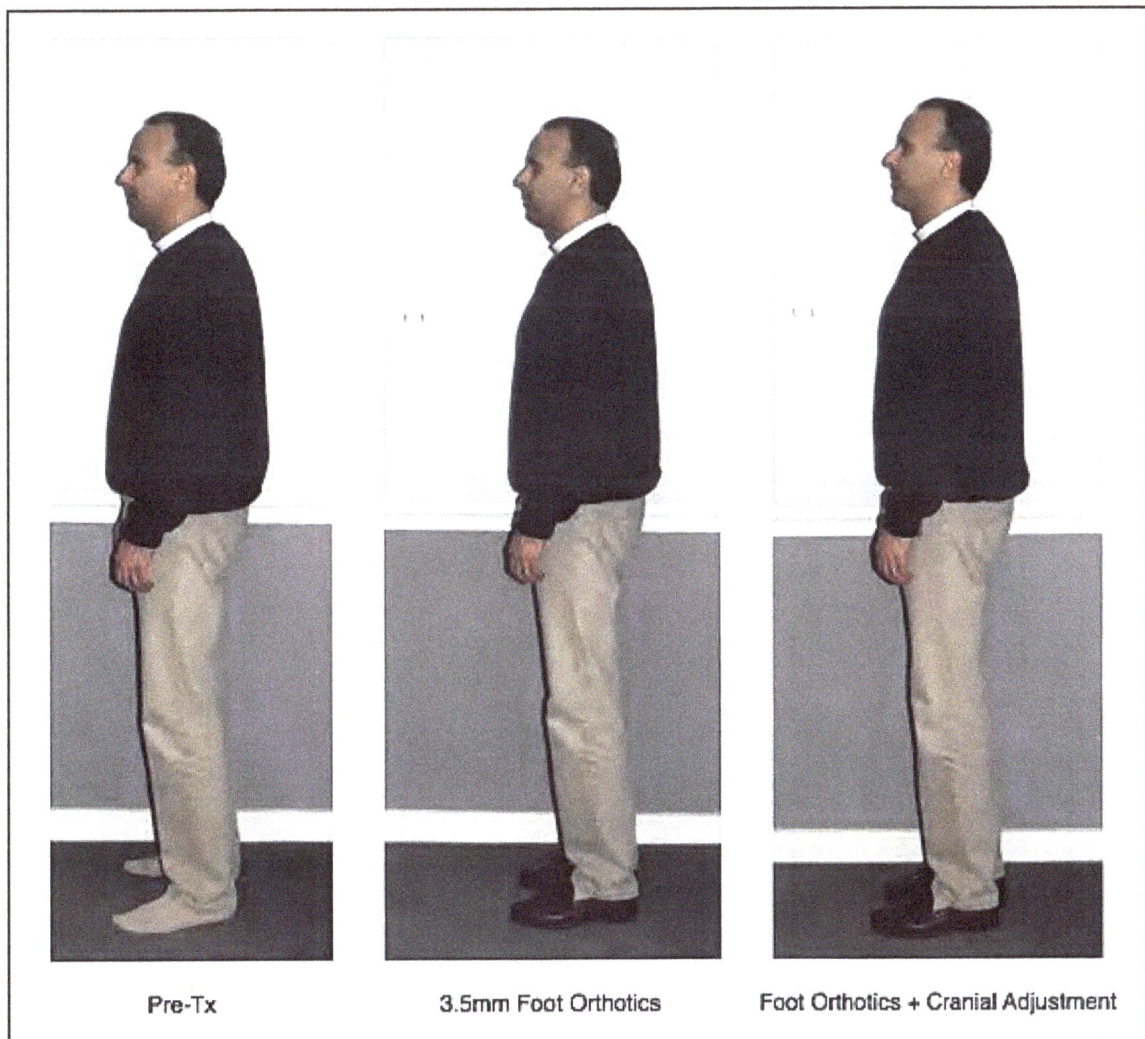

| Pre-Tx | 3.5mm Foot Orthotics | Foot Orthotics + Cranial Adjustment |

Treatment involved cranial adjustment, orthotics to correct foot alignment, and a resin bonded shim on the lower left second molar to support the cranium.

It is said that pictures express a thousand words. The following three photographs were taken December 6, 2012 before treatment, immediately after the foot orthotics were inserted, and immediately after the cranial adjustment was performed. Left side posterior occlusal contact was greatly improved by placement of a resin shim on the second molar tooth.

Dental, Cervical, Shoulder, Pelvic Pain Connection

Out of pure frustration, Guilherme Monteiro flew in from Australia to seek help in resolving his chronic neck, shoulder, and pelvic pain. He was evaluated by many dentists, chiropractors, and physicians with no result. He did experience some relief when a dental orthotic appliance was fabricated to increase the vertical height between his jaws. Unfortunately, no one had any answers on how to resolve his issues.

A comprehensive examination revealed multiple factors that were contributing to his pain pattern. First, he had a cranial structural distortion that no one picked up. This distortion caused a torquing or twisting of his dural membrane system in his skull and all the way down his spine. The increased tension in his dural tube was the underlying reason for the neck, shoulder, and pelvic pain. When upper and lower ALF appliances were inserted and adjusted to correct the cranial distortions, Guilherme's pain was reduced by 90 percent.

Overlying his structural problem was the presence of an underactive thyroid. His hypothyroidism was caused by an accumulation of heavy metals in his thyroid-lead, mercury, cadmium, arsenic, and nickel. In addition, there was cytomegalovirus (CMV) and Epstein-Barr virus (EBV) in his thyroid and the EBV was also in his upper left first molar, which had previously been treated with a root canal procedure. The EBV virus had also drained into his left tonsil. Guilherme also had glyphosate (Monsanto's herbicide, Round-Up), hepatitis B, and smallpox vaccine in his thyroid. These findings can only be determined by energetic testing because the substances were trapped within organs (thyroid, tooth, and tonsil) and will not show up in any blood test. For this reason, it is my professional opinion that blood tests have a very limited ability to determine what is wrong with a patient.

Guilherme's treatment was a long-term process. First, a nutritional program was set up to cleanse his liver. Following this, nutrients were provided to chelate the heavy metals, pesticide, and to support the immune system to resolve the CMV and EBV pathogens.

The last issues to be detoxed are the hepatitis B and small pox vaccines, which can be neutralized by the use of nosodes (homeopathic remedies made from the actual vaccine).

Most chronic cases have a multitude of underlying factors that traditional dentistry and medicine are not aware of. Complex problems require a complex treatment approach.

Treating symptoms with drugs and/or nutrients is not getting to the root cause. Unfortunately, the paradigm on which traditional dentistry and medicine is built is based on false science.

The x-ray (below) of the upper left second molar (root canal tooth) reveals a shadow around the roots. Energetic testing revealed Epstein-Barr virus in this tooth, which is the toxic waste dump feeding the tonsils and thyroid. The lymphatic or drainage system transports all toxic materials from the teeth and mouth to the thyroid and thymus glands and then throughout the rest of the body. When these toxins become concentrated enough, they can trigger a disease.

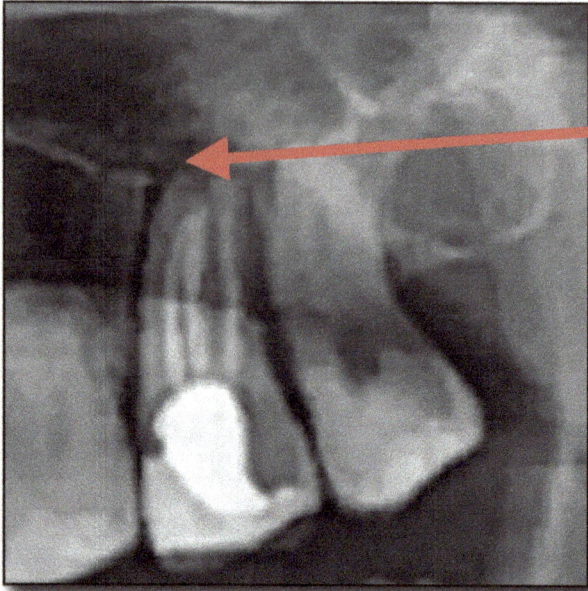

Toxic Microorganisms in Root Canal Treated Teeth (Hal Huggins, D.D.S., M.S.)

"Our first DNA studies examined bacteria retrieved from crushed root tips. We can identify eighty-three different anaerobic bacterial species with DNA testing. Root canal teeth contain fifty-three different species out of these eighty-three samples. Some are more dangerous than others, and some occur frequently, some occasionally. Selecting those that occur more than 5% of the time, we found:

• Capnocytophaga ochracea
• Fusobacterium nucleatum
• Gemella morbillorum
• Leptotrichia buccalis
• Porphyromonas gingivalis"

Of what significance are these? Four affect the heart, three the nerves, two the kidneys, two the brain, and one the sinus cavities. Shouldn't we question the wisdom of supplying a haven for these microbes that are so close to or in our brain and circulatory system? Does this information validate the claims of "sterile" root canals?

Dentists claim they can "sterilize" the tooth before forcing the gutta percha wax down into the canal. Perhaps they can sterilize a column of air in the center of the tooth, but is that really where the problem is? Bacteria wandering out of the dentinal tubules is what Weston A. Price, D.D.S. was finding, and what we were finding in the crushed tooth samples. But does the problem end there? Hardly.

Just out of curiosity, we tested blood samples adjacent to the removed teeth and analyzed them for the presence of anaerobic bacteria. Approximately 400 percent more bacteria were found in the blood surrounding the root canal tooth than were in the tooth itself. It seems that the tooth is the incubator. The periodontal ligament supplies more food and therefore a higher concentration of bacteria.

But the winner in pathological growth was in the bone surrounding the dead tooth. Looking at bacterial needs, there is a smorgasbord of bacterial nutrients present in the bone. This explains the tremendous increase in bacterial concentration in the blood surrounding the root canal tooth. Try sterilizing that volume of bone.

(Root Canal Dangers JUNE 25, 2010 BY HAL HUGGINS, D.D.S., M.S.)

The dental profession has been aware of Weston A. Price's research regarding the toxicity of root canal teeth since 1910. Unfortunately, the American Dental Association has adopted Joseph Goebbels' philosophy, "If you tell a big lie long enough and keep repeating it, people will eventually come to believe it."

The human body is like a "slinky." If you place a distortion at one end it will travel down to the other end. Medicine and dentistry have no understanding of the concept of functional anatomy. Their paradigm focuses primarily on treating symptoms. Practitioners must start viewing the body from a global perspective in order to understand that no matter how small an issue is affecting the body, it will impact on the entire organism.

Physiologic Complex
The Basis of Our Health

If one embarks on a project to build a house, the first thing that must be done is to level the foundation. One of the foundations of the human body is the cell membrane. If this structure is not functioning properly, the whole system will fail. The biggest assault on our cell membrane is coming from the food and vitamin industries. The processed, adulterated fats used in cooking (adulterated omega-6 oils: safflower, sunflower, corn, soy, and canola) and prepared foods are corrupting our cell membranes. These corrupted fats are literally converting the cell membranes into plastic. This impermeable membrane is one of the basic factors in the decline of our health (diabetes, cancer, macular degeneration, and cardiovascular disease).

The second destructive factor is fish oils, which is actually anti-freeze for fish. When fish swim in thirty degree water, the oil prevents them from freezing. The problem with fish oil is that at room temperature, 70 degrees Fahrenheit, it becomes rancid. At body temperature, 98.6 degrees Fahrenheit, the fish oil becomes completely rancid. This is the reason patients burp and belch and do not feel so good after ingesting it.

Fats Your Doctor Will Never Tell You About
Rebuilding the Cell Membrane

Most practitioners are well meaning but their knowledge base is at minimum twenty years behind the research. They prescribe supplements without understanding the physiology or the mechanism of how they work in the cell wall. The vitamin and pharmaceutical industries have spent millions of dollars to disseminate disinformation. It took approximately ten years to convince doctors to prescribe fish oils. Scientifically, it has been documented that fish oils corrupt the mitochondria of the heart and all cell membranes, preventing oxygen from getting in and waste products from getting out.

The cell wall is made up of half protein and half fats. Of the half fat portion, 50% or one quarter is saturated fats, which are nonreactive, and 50% or one quarter is unsaturated fats. The cell wall requires Parent Essential Oils (PEOs) to function properly. Unfortunately, many so-called essential fatty acids are really derivatives of the Parent Essential Oils. The only two Parent Essential Oils are omega-6 (linoleic acid) and the Parent omega-3 (alpha-linolenic acid). The term "Parent" is used because these are the whole, unadulterated, fully functional forms as they occur in nature and the only two essential fats your body requires. From these two PEOs the body can make the docosahexaenoic acid (DHA) and eicosapentaenoic acid (EPA) and other derivatives required by the brain and other organs and tissues.

According to Professor Brian S. Peskin, BSEE-MIT, Founder of Life-Systems Engineering Science, once the PEO's are consumed, your body changes a small percentage – less than 1% – into other biochemical entities called "derivatives," while leaving the remaining 99% in parent form. State-of-the-art 21st century analysis with positron emission testing (PET) proves this fact. Twenty-five to thirty-three percent (25%-33%) of every cell membrane's lipids are supposed to be PEO's (primarily omega-6s), which make up the bricks and mortar of the membrane. The brain only needs 7.2 milligrams per day of DHA and EPA to function, and the half-life of these oils in the brain is 2.5 years. This figure was established by scientific research by the National Institutes of Health and the U.S. Department of Agriculture.

Physicians who recommend taking 1000 mg of fish oil are doing irreparable damage to their patients. Fish oils are processed to remove their foul odor and increase their shelflife. The fish oils in cold-water fish act as antifreeze. Verification is derived from the fact that warm water fish have 14 times less fish oil than their cold water counterparts. Fish oil turns rancid at 70 degrees fahrenheit, room temperature, and it takes eighteen weeks to get it out of your body. The whole industry started when they couldn't get rid of the spoiled fish so they juiced them and encapsulated their rancid oils. When the adulterated omega-6 oils get incorporated into the cell membranes, the amount of oxygen that passes through is greatly diminished. When the oxygen levels become decreased by 35%, the cells transition into disease, cancer, and death. The adulterated oils also prevent production of the needed derivatives DHA/EPA resulting in deficiencies and dysfunction.

Many physicians believe that cholesterol, especially low-density lipids (LDLs), is harmful. In reality, the LDLs transport the PEOs to where they are needed. Prescribing statin drugs to lower one's cholesterol (LDLs) deprives the body of needed cholesterol for hormone production, and brain repair, and low levels ultimately are detrimental to one's health. The Cliff Notes version is that statin drugs shrink your brain by decreasing your cholesterol levels. Since your brain is 70% cholesterol, reducing its availability prevents the brain from repairing itself, causing dementia. Also stains drugs (Lipitor, Crestor, Pravachol, Zocor, Livalo, Mevacor, and Lescol) cause type two diabetes, rhabdomyolysis (breakdown of muscle tissue), liver damage, kidney failure, insomnia, joint pain, urinary tract infections, nausea, diarrhea, cold symptoms, vomiting, stomach cramps, leg pains, muscle weakness, and memory loss. One precaution mentioned in the statin drug literature warns patients to avoid drinking grapefruit juice, since it may decrease the ability of your liver to metabolize some of the statin drugs.

Our body requires special fats that make it possible, among other important functions, for sufficient oxygen to reach the cells. These special fats are highly oxygen-absorbing, and are called EFAs. However, it is the PEOs – not the commonly erroneously termed EFAs – like EPA and DHA from fish oil – that are important.

Why are the parent forms, the PEOs, so important? Many of the EFAs sold in stores consist of concentrated/processed EFA derivatives. Our bodies don't need or want these overdoses of derivatives, because we make our own derivatives out of the PEOs we consume, as we need them. Thus, taking fish oil and other health food store "EFAs" often results in overdosing the patient with derivatives, which can be very harmful. However, PEOs are essential and must be supplied from outside the body every day, from foods and certain oils. Your body can't manufacture PEOs (genuine EFAs, rather than EFA derivatives) on its own.

Every one of our 80 to 100 trillion cells is surrounded by a bilipid thin membrane. The cell membrane is half fat. A portion of the fat making up the membrane is saturated. "Saturated" means chemically nonreactive – in other words, it doesn't easily react with, or absorb, the oxygen and other biologic substances that come into contact with it. The other portion of the fat in the membrane is, however, "unsaturated." It, on the other hand, easily absorbs oxygen.

One of the major functions of unsaturated or polyunsaturated fats (omega-6) in the cell membrane is to facilitate the passage of oxygen into our cells. The Parent omega-6, fatty acid in the cell membrane, acts as a cellular "oxygen magnet." Where these essential fats are absent in cellular membranes, cells starve for oxygen, – even if the blood is highly oxygenated. Lowering the oxygen level by one-third will result in fermentation (similar to the process required to make beer and wine) and ultimately result in the formation of cancer cells. The saturated fats in the membrane function as a barrier to help protect the delicate, highly reactive, oxygen-absorbing, energizing, unsaturated fats in the membrane–the Parent omega-6.

The brain and nervous system comprise only 3% of total body weight. There are normally only small, trace amounts of these EPA/DHA derivatives used in the brain, eyes, and nervous system in the plasma, cellular membranes, and tissues in the human body. Contrary to PEO requirements, extremely little is required for their daily replenishment. Marine and fish oil supplements in their suggested dosages, however, supply EPA and DHA in supraphysiologic amounts, often in excess of 100-fold, or even 500-fold more than the body would ever naturally produce on its own.

Because the fish oil is the source of the EPA and DHA, these oils are rancid, and the body has to divert anti-oxidants to counteract these toxic, adulterated oils.

It is wrong to recommend a derivative when the fully functional, unadulterated "Parent" Essential Oil" is required. Research demonstrates that fish oil supplements consistently fail to prevent cardiovascular disease, cancer, and significantly worsen diabetic patients' condition by raising blood sugar levels and lessening the critical insulin response.

Most cooking oils are based on Parent omega-6 oils and food processors adulterate these oils (for longer shelf-life), making them no longer oxygen-absorbing or fully functional. One hundred trillion (100,000,000,000) defective cell membranes would be expected to cause enormous health problems–and they do–from cardiovascular disease, to cancer, to diabetes.

Many cardiologists recommend that patients take aspirin on a daily basis to prevent blood clots and a heart attack. Although aspirin does thin the blood, it also corrupts the omega-6 oils in the cell membranes, which thus interferes with oxygen absorption and prevents production of the essential derivative oils. Routine use of aspirin or other NSAIDs (non-steroidal anti-inflammatory drugs) not only prevents the uptake of amino acids to repair arthritic joints but also the leading cause of gastric bleeding. These issues are easily remedied by taking Co enzyme Q10 or systemic enzymes like Zymessence to prevent clots.

Methyl Sulfonyl Methane (MSM)

MSM is classified by the FDA as a food. It supplies 35% organic sulfur. Sulfur is the third most prevalent mineral in the body. Some people may react to sulfur, sulfates, or sulfides. However the sulfonyl form of sulfur in MSM is not one of the forms that people are "allergic" to. One key factor about this organic sulfur is that it helps repair the cell membranes. Half of the cell membrane is composed of protein.

When incorporated into the protein portion of the membrane, organic sulfur restores flexibility to the structure. This makes the membrane more permeable, allowing nutrients to enter the cell more easily and waste products to exit more efficiently. Increasing a cell membrane's permeability is a major factor in reversing the aging process. One can take the best quality nutrients on this planet, but if they cannot get into the cell they are of little use. Using MSM must be an essential part of any therapy when treating all types of disease. Toxicity from what- ever source along with the wrong fats and lack of organic sulfur corrupt the membranes throughout the body and provide the basis for disease.

Systemic Enzymes

The disease process has the following progression: irritation, inflammation, fibrosis, dysfunction, disease, and death. The use of systemic enzymes is the one essential ingredient to help reduce and reverse not only disease but aging. One just has to realize that irritation can come from many potential sources. Heavy metals, pesticides, chemicals, bacteria, viruses, mold, funguses, metal implants, tattoos, scars, oral infections, hypothyroidism, insulin, carbohydrates (which raise insulin levels), breast implants, EMFs (electromagnetic frequencies), toxic intestines, constipation, wounds, and sunburn represent some of the common irritants that affect us.

After the age of 27, the pancreas decreases its production of pancreatic enzymes. It is these enzymes that control the fibrosis or scarring that is caused by inflammation. The older we get, the more scarring that occurs within our body and the reason we get stiffer as we age. In addition to dissolving away the scarring, systemic enzymes reduce inflammation throughout the body. They even clear the blood of any foreign protein that may be present. They also work as an effective antibiotic, destroying bacteria, and they are mildly effective as an anti-viral agent. Systemic enzymes work to clear the plaque from the blood vessels, remove the fibrosis from organs, and increase microcirculation throughout the body, restoring the body to a younger physiologic age.

Dr. William Wong stated, "Systemic enzymes are the most important part of maintaining a healthy body; of fighting the processes of both aging and disease; and of undoing the planned obsolescence nature has built into our bodies to make sure we don't stay on the planet for too long.

Systemic enzymes are the only nontoxic way of controlling inflammation of every type and for whatever reason. More importantly, they are the only tools available in both natural and allopathic ("conventional") medicine for fighting fibrosis. We have to remember that most all disease names end with one of two suffixes, either the "itis" denoting an inflammation or an "osis" denoting a fibrosis condition. Most of what winds up killing people is either an inflammation (itis), such as heart and vascular disease, diabetes, cancer, trauma, Alzheimer's disease, or a fibrosis (osis) related event such as a clot-caused stroke or heart attack; fibrosis of the kidney, liver, or heart valves; or age related shrinking of the internal organs. We also have to remember that of the two diseases that cause fibrosis, inflammation is the number one major reaction that brings about the formation of fibrosis and scar tissue. So control the one and you prevent the further formation of the other."
(Zymessence: The New Breed of Systemic Enzyme Blends. By: William Wong ND, PhD, Member of the World Sports Medicine Hall of Fame)

There are many systemic enzyme products on the market; however, the best one is Zymessence, which was formulated by Dr. William Wong. It is a pharmaceutical grade serrapeptase that istwelve tosixteen times more potent than chymotrypsin. Chymotrypsin is one of the pancreatic enzymes that was used by Drs. William B. Kelly and Nicholas Gonzalez. Both practitioners had an 85% success rate in treating pancreatic cancer. The effectiveness of this systemic enzyme is due to the fact that it can dissolve away the biofilm that cancer cells secret to protect themselves from the body's own immune system. It also has the ability to dissolve cancer cells.

Synergy of Nutrients

Nothing works alone. The minerals need the vitamins, and both require the enzymes to fully function. The systemic enzymes mentioned above work globally within the body as an anti-inflammatory, to dissolve fibrin (scars), digest foreign protein in the blood, and they are bactericidal and mildly antiviral. The Zymessence is double enteric coated so it does not get destroyed by stomach acids and works in the alkaline environment of the small intestines. In contrast, plant enzymes have a broader pH range in which they work. They work efficiently both in the stomach and small intestines because they have a functional pH range of 3 to 9; they work in both an acidic and alkaline environment. The optimal temperature range for most plant enzymes is 92°F to 104°F, which means that these enzymes work best at body temperature. Cooking, baking, microwaving, canning, and pasteurizing occur above 118⁰F and destroy the plant enzymes. Shipment from the growing source to consumer location also takes its toll and greatly reduces their potency or totally destroys them. The purpose of the food enzymes is mainly to digest food, but they also have some anti-inflammatory properties, as evidenced in bromelain and papain. In general, patients with hypothyroidism have a low body temperature, which directly affects the function of plant enzymes and is one of the reasons these patients have poor digestion.

Your Gut Accounts for 60% to 80% of Your Immune System

Another major component of the immune system is the gut. The approximately 25 to 30 feet of intestines provide a home to billions of microorganisms, which provide the basis for 60% to 80% of our immune system. Multiple sources that have the potential to corrupt our microbiome are: sugar, chemicals, rancid oils, electromagnetic frequencies (wi-fi and microwaves), antibiotics, most medications, processed foods, herbicides (especially glyphosate), and steroids. In addition, our gut directly links to our brain via the lymphatic system and the tenth or vagus nerve. People with toxic guts invariably run into early dementia and other neurological issues. Beside cleaning up the diet by eating organic foods, one should provide a good pre and probiotic supplement. In my practice, I use primarily, Bravo yogurt (from Switzerland) and Prescript-Assist to repopulate the intestines.

The thyroid gland plays a major role in the functioning of your immune system. From my clinical experience, blood tests are not a good indicator to determine if it is working. Twenty years of research by Dr. Broda Barnes showed that your armpit temperature plus clinical symptoms are the best diagnostic indicators to determine if an under or overactive thyroid exists. Clinically, I have found that the childhood vaccines, especially tetanus are being trapped in the left lobe of the thyroid. I have also observed that herbicides (especially glyphosate), mercury, and cytomegalovirus also get trapped within the left lobe of the thyroid. Treatment involves removing the offending items, with nutrients, to assist the organ to function properly. Just shotgunning standard protocol such as iodine or desiccated thyroid is a losing battle to restore normalcy.

Liver Transplant Averted by Defining The "Splinters"

The title, *Remove the "Splinters"and Watch the Body Heal*, defines the paradigm formulated by this author. After fifty years of clinical practice, I came to the realization that blood tests and most other diagnostic testing used by allopathic or conventional medicine are not accurate. For the most part, all the testing accomplishes is "analysis paralysis." The doctors have so many test results, but they have not connected the dots. Because they are at a loss for the underlying cause, their only option is surgery or drugs. Traditional testing for the most part does not tell you the underlying cause of the patient's problem. Case in point: In 2011, Fred Schmidt came to my office because he was told he needed a liver transplant. He had suffered from a swollen liver for 27 years, and no medical testing had been able to decipher the cause. Not happy with the prognosis and idea that he would be on steroids for the rest of his life, Fred decided to get another opinion. In one hour, using Quantum Testing, it was determined that the reason for Fred's swollen liver and elevated alkaline phosphatase level was the presence of benzene and hepatitis B in his liver.

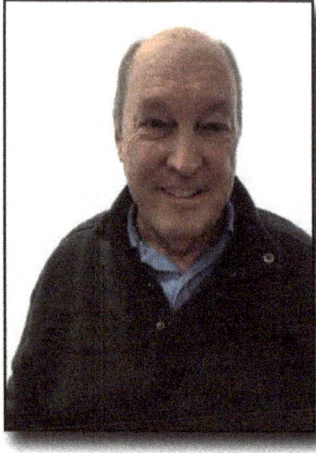

Fred was placed on a nutritional program to remove the two "splinters." In seven months, Fred's liver went back to "factory default," and his alkaline phosphatase level also normalized. For the past nine years Fred's blood tests have all been normal but his insurance company still will not insure him. Fred has a normal liver and is a happy camper. In my opinion, medicine's tool box is obsolete and needs a serious upgrade.

The case studies that have been presented in this book and the ones to follow are offered to further illustrate the need to look for the cause and not just the abnormal blood values.

What Eczema, Insomnia, Weight Gain, Fatigue, Anxiety, and Depression All Have in Common

Aditi was referred to my office for chronic, severe eczema, insomnia, weight gain, fatigue, lack of zest for life, anxiety and depression, and upper neck pain. She had been evaluated by many conventional physicians and even naturopathic practitioners with no resolution of her chief complaints. This medical journey went on for several years, and Aditi became very frustrated. Because the conventional diagnostics failed to uncover the causes of her issues, Quantum Testing Technique (QTT) was used. This latest technology detects energy imbalances years before abnormal clinical signs and blood indicators appear. The QTT revealed several major stressors: heavy metals, herbicides, viruses, hypothyroidism, and hypoadrenia were present. This advanced technology is incredibly accurate and represents the next generation of advanced technology to be used in the practice of quantum medicine.

Once the underlying offending stressors were discovered, Aditi was placed on a specific nutritional program to remove them. The key to successful treatment is simple: diagnose and then remove the initiators of the disease process by giving the body the appropriate food-based supplementation. The healing begins, and the symptoms disappear. The conventional model being used at present is obsolete and unable to detect the etiology of the patient's problem. Present-day medicine is wrapped up in analysis paralysis, that is, practitioners have volumes of test results but they are still unable to connect the dots and discover the causes.

Following the initial visit in August of 2017, Aditi returned in three months. Although they were not totally gone, her symptoms were definitely reduced. A re-evaluation was performed, and her supplement program was adjusted. Aditi returned for a six month re-evaluation visit and was a very happy camper. Her progress was incredible: Her chronic severe eczema was totally gone; her insomnia was nonexistent; she had lost 16 pounds; she stated that she was like the energizer bunny with a renewed zest for life; and she experienced no more anxiety and depression. Also of interest was the fact that she stated that her neck pain had totally resolved following her first visit when a comprehensive cranial adjustment was performed. The accompanying photographs tell the story, along with the video testimonial.

Pre-TX Images

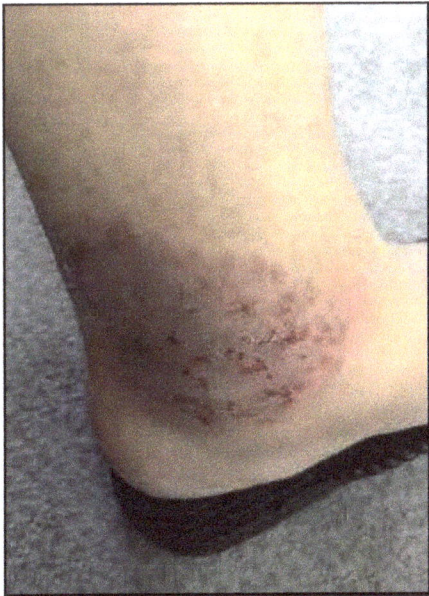 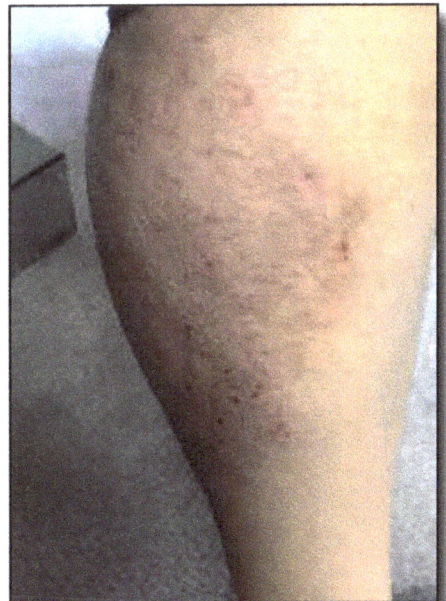

Post-TX Images

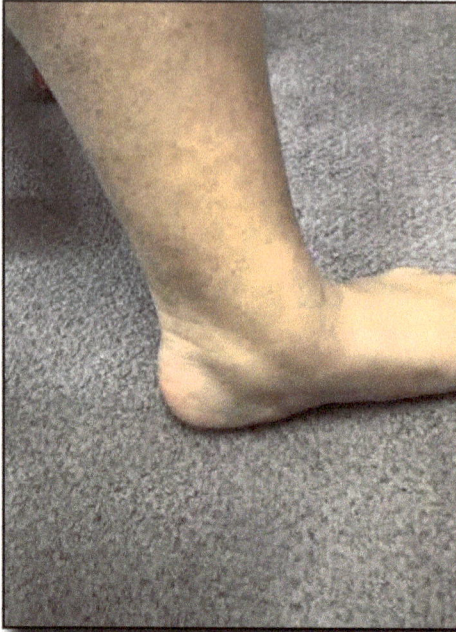

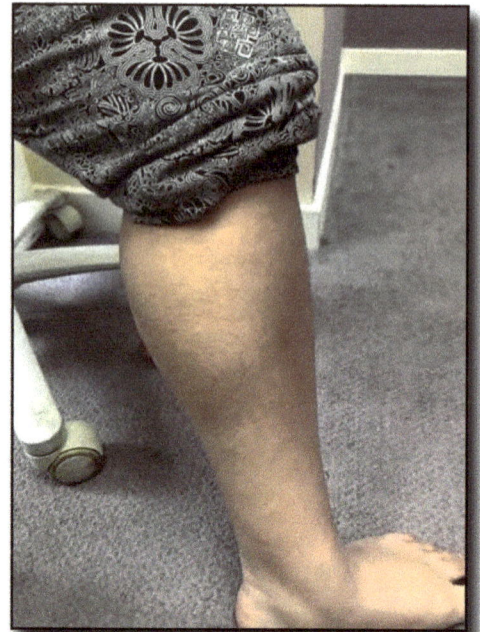

Follow-up treatment was provided with the Bioptron I System (full spectrum light), which has removed the remaining discoloration.

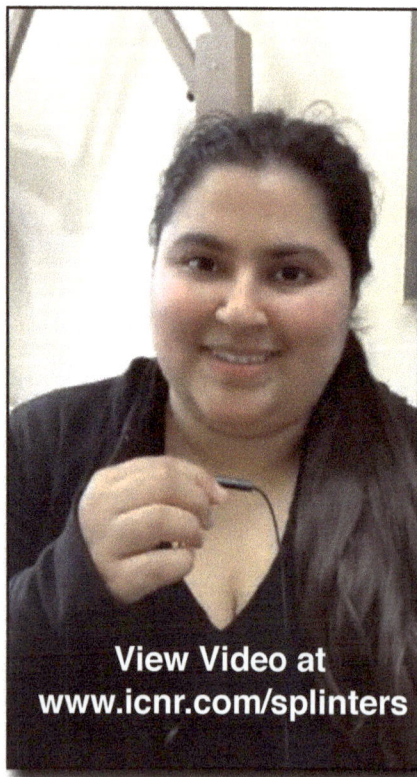

View Video at
www.icnr.com/splinters

Parasite Treatment

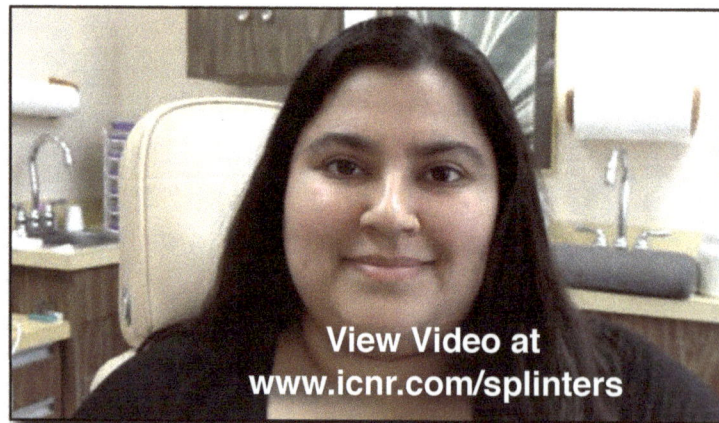

View Video at
www.icnr.com/splinters

Eczema Treatment

Approximately a year after resolving her severe eczema, Aditi developed another set of complaints of floaters in her eyes and a sharp low back pain. Quantum Testing diagnosed intestinal parasites. In just two treatments with ivermectin two weeks apart, Aditi's symptoms of both the floaters and the low back pain disappeared. Using the Quantum Testing protocol is like a laser guided bomb - extremely accurate in finding its target.

The skin is the second biggest excretory system of the body. When the liver, kidneys, lungs, spleen, and intestines cannot handle the wastes, they are excreted through the surface of the skin. If the toxins are relatively benign, they appear as pimples, blisters, or rashes. If the toxic substances are adulterated omega-6 oils, there is a high probability that they will cause skin cancer. It is not the ultraviolet A or ultraviolet B spectrum of the light that causes skin cancer, but the corrupted oils that get trapped and reduced oxygenation of the cells.

Say no to or carefully research medical drugs. One of the conventional treatments for eczema is the use of Humira. One must approach the use of drugs with caution. First, is the body deficient in the medication being prescribed? Second, what are its potential side effects? Third, is there a safer alternative to drug therapy? For the majority of natural remedies, there are NO side effects. Remember, your physician is not well versed in natural remedies and will not offer another option.

Please take the time to review the side effects of Humira before taking a leap of faith.

Common side effects of Humira include: upper respiratory tract infection, headache, injection site reaction, skin rash, antibody development, sinusitis, and pain at injection site. Other side effects include: urinary tract infection, abdominal pain, and flu-like symptoms. See below for a comprehensive list of the 103 adverse effects of this medication.

More Common Side Effects:

Body aches or pain	Nasal congestion
Ear congestion	Pain or tenderness around the eyes or cheekbones
Cough	Rapid and sometimes shallow breathing
Gas with abdominal or stomach pain	Shivering
Hoarseness	Stomach fullness
Lightheadedness	Sunken eyes
Loss of voice	Thirst
Lower back or side pain	Trouble sleeping
Muscle aches and pains	Warmth on the skin
	Wrinkled skin

Less Common:

Abnormal vaginal bleeding or discharge	Lump in the breast or under your arm
Agitation	Lump or swelling in the abdomen or stomach
Arm, back, or jaw pain	Mole that leaks fluid or bleeds
Black, tarry stools	Muscle cramps or spasms
Bleeding from the gums or nose	Nausea
Blindness	New mole
Bloating or swelling of the face, arms, hands, lower legs, or feet	Night sweats
Blood in the stool or change in bowel habits	No blood pressure or pulse
Bloody or cloudy urine	Noisy breathing
Blurred vision	Numbness or tingling in your arms, legs, or face
broken bones	Pain, redness, or swelling in the arms or legs without any injury present
Change in size, shape, or color of an existing mole	Pale skin
Change in skin color	Persistent non-healing sore on your skin
Chest pain, tightness, or heaviness	Pink growth

Chills	Puffiness or swelling of the eyelids or around the eyes, face, lips, or tongue
Clear or bloody discharge from the nipple	Raised, firm, or bright red patch
Cold hands and feet	Redness or swelling of the breast
Confusion	Seeing or hearing things that are not there
Constipation	Seizures
Cough	Sharp back pain just below your ribs
Coughing or spitting up blood	Shiny bump on your skin
Decreased urination	Slurred speech or problems with swallowing
Decreased vision	Sneezing
Depression	Sore on the skin of the breast that does not heal
difficulty with breathing	sore throat
Difficult, burning, or painful urination	Sores, ulcers, or white spots on the lips or mouth
Dimpling of the breast skin	Spitting up blood
Dizziness	Stiff neck
Drowsiness	Stomach pain
Eye pain	Stopping of the heart
Fainting	Sudden high fever or low grade fever for months
Fast, slow, or irregular heartbeat	Sweating
Fever	Swelling of the face, fingers, feet, or lower legs
Forgetfulness	Swollen glands
Frequent urge to urinate	Swollen neck veins
General feeling of illness	Tiredness
Hair loss	Trouble breathing with activity
Headache	Trouble thinking
Increased thirst	Unconsciousness
Inverted nipple	Unexplained bruising or bleeding
Irregular breathing	Unpleasant breath odor
Irregular pulse	Unusual tiredness or weakness

irritability	Unusual weight gain or loss
Itching or rash	Visual disturbances
Light colored stools	Vomiting
Loss of appetite	Vomiting of blood or material that looks like coffee grounds
	Yellow skin or eyes

"Never trust a doctor who has dying plants in his or her reception room."
Author unknown

Drug-Induced Vertigo

For the past thirty years, Carmen M. has had tubes in his ear canals to keep his Eustachian tubes open. In 2017, he developed an infection in his left ear. The ENT

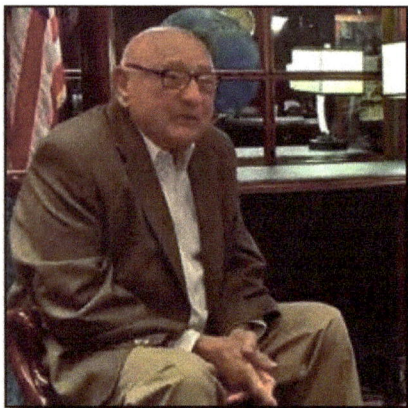

physician prescribed the drug Ciprodex®, which is a combination of an antibiotic and a steroid. Within ten minutes after the Ciprodex® was placed in Carmen's left ear, he developed vertigo. How many double blind studies and tests does one have to perform to substantiate the connection between the drug and the cause of the vertigo? For over a year, Carmen was examined by top neurologists, ENT physicians, and had numerous tests performed. All the gold standard procedures failed to diagnose and resolve Carmen's vertigo.

Carmen's son brought his father in my office for an evaluation. Of additional interest, was the fact that Carmen presented with a deep overbite (loss of vertical height), which was the underlying cause for his need of Eustachian tubes. If Carmen's bite had been corrected thirty years ago, he would not have needed the ear tubes. During the course of my medical history taking, the information was obtained regarding the use of Ciprodex®. I requested that the patient bring the drug into my office at his next visit. A cranial adjustment was performed to correct an existing structural distortion. The patient did experience some relief of his vertigo during the next several weeks.

On the second visit, the Ciprodex® was energetically tested and found to be trapped in the auditory nerve in his left ear. What traditional medicine does not understand is that the use of drugs has another major downside: the chemicals in the formula have the potential of becoming trapped within tissues like nerves and organs. A homeopathic remedy was energetically made from the actual drug. The patient was instructed to take nine drops under his tongue three times a day between meals. Of interest:, Carmen has NOT had a bout of vertigo since starting the homeopathic remedy. Does anyone doubt the drug-vertigo connection or the efficacy of using homeopathic remedies?

Of historical interest, the Royal Family of England has a homeopathic physician, Dr. Peter Fisher. He is Clinical Director and Director of Research at the Royal London Hospital for Integrated Medicine. Doctor Fisher has stated that homeopathy is "safe," "popular with patients,' and has reduced the need for antibiotics. What an interesting comment to be made particularly in light of the fact that our own Food and Drug Administration is in the process of eliminating the use of homeopathy in our country because it interferes with Big Pharma's profits.

The unfortunate state of affairs in the U.S. is that more people would call their congress representative if the telecast of the Superbowl was cancelled than if their right to have access to homeopathics was being taken away by the FDA.

What are the possible side effects of CIPRODEX® otic?
CIPRODEX® otic may cause serious side effects. Stop using this drug and call your doctor if you have any of the following signs or symptoms of: allergic reactions;

hives; trouble breathing; swelling of your face, lips, mouth, or tongue; rash; itching; dizziness; fast heartbeat; pounding in your chest.

IMPORTANT! You should not use Ciprodex® ear drops if you have a viral infection that is affecting your ear canal, including herpes or chicken pox.

Depression, Panic Attacks, and Anxiety Linked to Thyroid

Depression is the leading cause for disability worldwide. As with most medical issues, there are multiple factors for the underlying cause(s). Because blood tests to assess thyroid function are inaccurate, thyroid dysfunction is frequently overlooked in the diagnosis of depression. Remember that blood tests only detect the thyroid hormones in the blood and not in the cells. Broda Barnes' twenty years of research on hypothyroidism documented that a patient's symptoms coupled with armpit temperature was the best way to determine an underactive thyroid.

In addition to depression there, is a long list of symptoms associated with hypothyroidism:

Anxiety	Mental fog
Panic Attacks	Enlarged heart
Insomnia	Muscle spasms
Heart palpitations	Ligament weakness
Dizziness	Cold hands and feet
Tinnitus (ear ringing)	Intolerance to cold
Digestion problems	Constipation
Thinning of the Hair	Poor memory
Dry skin	Poor reading comprehension
Brittle nails	Chronic pain (fibromyalgia)
Translucent skin	Inability to sweat
Acne	Weak immune system
Allergies	Fatigue, exhaustion

Butterfly rash over the bridge of the nose	Apathy
Increase tooth decay	Feeling of insecurity

A diagnosis can easily be confirmed by taking one's armpit temperature first thing in the morning before getting out of bed. If the reading is consistently below 97.8^0 F. over a period of one month, and many of the above symptoms are present, then the person has an underactive thyroid. Once a baseline temperature and diagnosis are established, the practitioner must determine what's in the thyroid that is preventing it from working. The causes can be many. Most often they involve mercury and other heavy metals, pesticides, chemicals (chlorine, bromide, fluoride), viruses, vaccines and adjuvants trapped in the thyroid, infections from a dental source (third molar extraction sites, root canal teeth, and toxic dental materials), and parasites. After diagnosing the cause then the appropriate remedies must be determined.

Once the offending "splinters" or initiators are removed, the thyroid starts functioning normally, and the symptoms will lessen or disappear. This was the case with Dr. J. Once her mercury levels were reduced in her thyroid, her depression, panic attacks, and anxiety totally disappeared. Taking medication such as antidepressants to mask the depression, panic attacks, and anxiety will only serve to make the problem worse over time.

Hear Dr. J's Testimonial at www.icnr.com/splvideo/

The Underlying Cause for Autoimmune Diseases

I honestly believe this label was conjured up by the medical establishment to cover-up their lack of knowledge and their Neanderthal mentality on how the body works. Just think about this for a moment. Why would the body in its infinite wisdom attack a healthy organ? In reality, there is some "splinter" within the organ that is causing the autoimmune system to kick in. The problem is that conventional medicine does not have the sophisticated technology to diagnose the initiator(s). This is where quantum physics runs circles around "conventional" medical testing.

The autoimmune scam first came to my attention in 2009 when my own daughter was diagnosed with Hashimoto's disease, an alleged autoimmune disease. Her endocrinologist wanted to prescribe Tapazole to suppress my daughter's overactive thyroid. I looked up the side effects of this drug.

Common Side Effects of Tapazole Include:

Stomach upset,	Drowsiness,
Nausea,	Dizziness,
Vomiting,	Muscle/joint/nerve pain,
Mild skin rash/itching,	Swelling, or
Headache,	Hair loss.

After I reviewed these potential issues, I told my daughter to tell her endocrinologist I would treat her with alternative therapies. He emphatically told her they would not work. Using Quantum Testing techniques, I diagnosed that Lori's thyroid gland had Epstein-Barr virus (EBV) trapped in it. Interestingly, my daughter had EBV when she was in her senior year of high school back in 1996. She spent 12 to 16 hours a day in bed because she was exhausted. Six doctors later we discovered she had EBV, which was reversed with homeopathic remedies. Fast forward to 2009;

the two remedies that tested positive against her Epstein-Barr virus were noni and colloidal silver. In addition, I loaned her my bio-frequency machine, which literally has the capability of exploding viruses without damaging any other tissues or organisms. Three months later all her endocrinologist's blood tests were normal, and he never called to find out what I did. There are no worse crimes on this planet than bruising a physician's ego.

The lesson to be learned from this event was that viruses never go away. They just lie dormant until some stressful event lowers the immune system, and they resurface. The key to staying healthy is eat clean and organic whenever possible, be happy, hug a tree once a week, take good quality food-based supplements, get enough sleep, drink clean filtered water, and say no to drugs.

The Mayo Clinic states that "Hashimoto's disease is the most common cause of hypothyroidism in the United States. It primarily affects middle-aged women but also can occur in men and women of any age and in children. Patients with Hashimoto's disease often first experience hyperthyroidism. With hyperthyroidism comes a high T4 (tetraiodothyronine), or T3 (triiodothyronine) level, both can cause an excessively high metabolic rate. This is called a hypermetabolic state. When a hypermetabolic state exists, you may experience a rapid heart rate, elevated blood pressure, and hand tremors. You may also sweat a lot and develop a low tolerance for heat. Hyperthyroidism can cause more frequent bowel movements, weight loss, and, in women, irregular menstrual cycles. Visibly, the thyroid gland can enlarge into a goiter, which can be either bilaterally swollen or one-sided. Your eyes may also appear quite prominent, which is a sign of exophthalmos, a condition that's related to Graves' disease.

Following a period of overactivity, and then a state of underactivity, hypothyroidism, follows. Hypothyroidism is associated with the following signs and symptoms:

Increase in tooth decay	Muscle weakness
A butterfly rash over the bridge of the nose	Excessive or prolonged menstrual bleeding (menorrhagia)
Appearance of acne	Depression
Fatigue and sluggishness	Memory lapses
Increased sensitivity to cold	Increased anxiety
Constipation	Loss of the lateral third of the eyebrow
Pale, dry skin	Infertility
Brittle nails	Insomnia
A puffy face	Weakened immune system: frequent colds
Thinning and Hair loss	Cold hands and feet
Enlargement of the tongue	Tinnitus or ringing of the ears
Unexplained weight gain	Palpitations of the heart
Muscle aches, tenderness and stiffness	Yellowish color to the soles of the feet
Joint pain and stiffness	

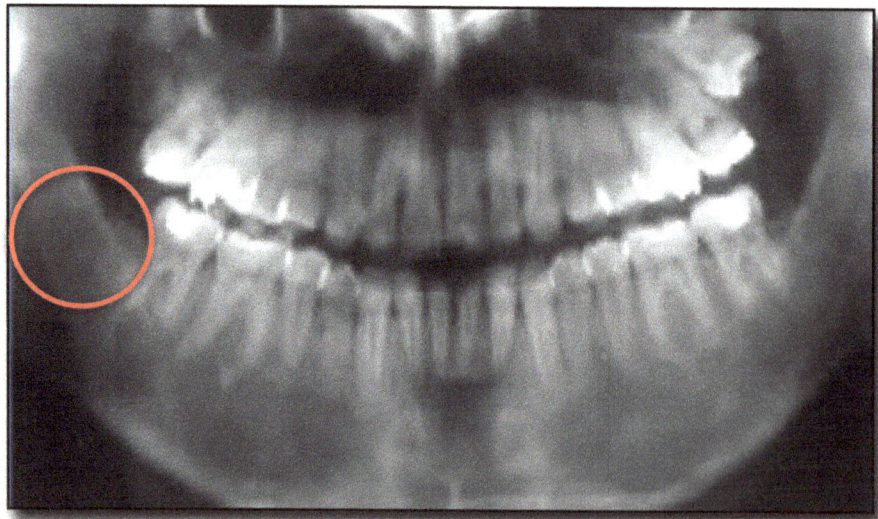

Hashimoto's Disease Revisited: The Dental Connection

The universe always has a way of testing you to see if your hypothesis is valid. Not too long after I successfully treated my daughter, one of my patients asked me if I would treat her daughter who was diagnosed with Hashimoto's disease.

Lisa was a 24-year-old accountant who was diagnosed with Hashimoto's disease by her medical doctor. Lisa presented with severe fatigue, weight gain, poor memory, and insomnia. When she came home from work, she would literally crash and have to go to bed.

My examination uncovered two key causative factors. One, was the presence of cytomegalovirus (CMV) in her jawbone where her lower right wisdom tooth had been extracted seven years before. The CMV had migrated via her lymphatic system into her thyroid. The second factor was nickel, which had its origin from a bonded orthodontic retaining wire behind her lower front teeth. The nickel ions also had migrated through her lymphatic system into her thyroid. Both the CMV and nickel were being attacked by her immune system. This was Lisa's source of her "autoimmune" disease. In reality, her immune system was doing its job. Unfortunately, the medical industry has no clue about these types of connections.

Cavitations are areas in the bone where a tooth was extracted and a residual infection remains. The red circle denotes the third molar post-extraction site where the cytomegalovirus resided. If you look closely, there is a thin horizontal line behind the lower front teeth where the orthodontic retaining wire was bonded to the teeth.

Lisa was placed on a nutritional program to combat the CMV infection and chelate out the nickel from her thyroid. Removal of the two offending items resulted in the disappearance of her "autoimmune" disease, along with her symptoms. In reality, there is no such thing as autoimmune disease. Practitioners must start looking for underlying causes if they are to be successful in their treatment.

Dental-Raynaud's Disease Connection

In my clinical experience since graduating dental school in 1969, I have come to the realization that 70% to 90% of all medical problems have a dental link and Raynaud's disease is no exception. The primary dental whole body connection comes from the direct effect of oral infections, toxic root canal teeth, leakage of mercury from mercury fillings, galvanic currents from mixed metals in the mouth, and the use of incompatible dental materials on the thyroid. Basic anatomy documents that ALL dental structures (gums, lips, tongue, jaw bone, floor of the mouth) are drained by the lymphatic tissue (sewage system of the body), which ultimately takes its contents through the thyroid gland. Once toxins are trapped in the thyroid, this endocrine gland becomes underactive.

It is this author's belief that many of the symptoms of Raynaud's disease are directly caused by an underactive thyroid, which lowers metabolism causing the body to automatically shunt blood away from the hands and feet in an attempt to raise the core body temperature. Exposure to cold exacerbates the condition because the body has to conserve heat. The muscle spasm associated with Raynaud's is directly caused by the muscle weakness caused by a low functioning thyroid. Although there are other potential causes for Raynaud's disease (see list below), my experience is that most cases are caused by an under-ctive thyroid, which is not being diagnosed because traditional blood tests ARE NOT SENSITIVE ENOUGH! Many Raynaud patients are suffering needlessly because of inaccurate testing procedures and failure of the physician to interpret the patient's cluster of symptoms common to hypothyroidism. Signs and symptoms of Raynaud's disease include: Cold fingers or toes. Color changes in your skin in response to cold or stress. Numb, prickly feeling or stinging pain upon warming or stress relief.

Case Study: Forty-Three Years of Suffering from Raynaud's Disease Resolved in Less than Two Weeks

One of my students who took a recent postgraduate seminar (October 2007), mentioned that she suffered from Raynaud's disease. As a dentist, she had numerous mercury fillings in her own mouth from childhood, and she also had excess exposure to mercury vapors from removing mercury fillings from patients throughout the years. She became burdened with mercury as a result of frequent exposure. The excess mercury became concentrated in her thyroid, resulting in hypothyroidism. She demonstrated many of the signs and symptoms listed on the Mayo Clinic's website for Raynaud's disease. The dentist also had an infection in her upper left second bicuspid tooth, which had undergone root canal therapy; this further burdened her thyroid. She was tested for the appropriate chelating nutrients and immune support for the infection, and in less than two weeks of therapy her Raynaud's symptoms disappeared.

The following description of Raynaud's disease appears on the Mayo Clinic's web site: www.mayoclinic.com.

Signs and Symptoms

"Raynaud's disease is more than simply having cold hands and cold feet, and it's not the same as frostbite. Signs and symptoms of Raynaud's depend on the frequency, duration and severity of the blood vessel spasms that underlie the disorder. Signs and symptoms include:

Sequence of color changes in your skin in response to cold or stress.

Numb, prickly feeling or stinging pain upon warming or relief of stress.

At first, during an attack of Raynaud's, the affected areas of your skin usually turn white. Then, the areas often turn blue and feel cold and numb, and your sensory perception is dull. The affected skin may look slightly swollen. As circulation improves, the affected areas may turn red, throb, and tingle or swell. The order of the changes of color isn't the same for all people, and not everyone experiences all three colors.

Occasionally, an attack affects just one or two fingers or toes. Attacks don't necessarily always affect the same digits. Although Raynaud's most commonly affects your fingers and toes, the condition can also affect other areas of your body such as your nose, cheeks, ears, and even tongue. An attack may last less than a minute to several hours. Over time, attacks may grow more severe.

Causes

Doctors don't completely understand the cause of Raynaud's attacks, but blood vessels in the hands and feet appear to overreact to cold temperatures or stress. *Editor's Note:* Any change in weather or physical activity will overburden an underactive thyroid.

When your body is exposed to cold temperatures, your extremities lose heat. Your body slows down the blood supply to your fingers and toes to preserve your body's core temperature. Your body specifically reduces blood flow by narrowing the small arteries under the skin of your extremities. In people with Raynaud's, this normal response is exaggerated. *Editor's Note:* The response is exaggerated because the body is already functioning below normal and any event that "threatens" unbalancing the body's homeostasis is met with an exaggerated response. Stress causes a similar reaction to cold in the body, and likewise the body's response may be exaggerated. *Editor's note:* Any stress to the body (physical, emotional, or chemical) will overburden an underactive thyroid.

With Raynaud's, arteries to your fingers and toes go into what's called vasospasm. This constricts the blood vessels, dramatically but temporarily limiting blood supply. Over time, these same small arteries may also thicken slightly, further limiting blood flow. The result is that affected skin turns a pale and dusky color due to the lack of blood flow to the area. Once the spasms subside and blood returns to the area, the tissue may turn red before returning to a normal pink color.

Cold temperatures are most likely to provoke an attack. Exposure to cold can be as simple as putting your hands under a faucet of running cold water, taking something out of the freezer or exposure to cold air. For some people, exposure to cold temperatures isn't necessary. Emotional stress alone can cause an episode of Raynaud's."

"Some researchers are studying whether Raynaud's may be partly an inherited disorder."

Primary Versus Secondary Raynaud's

Raynaud's disease occurs in two main types. Primary Raynaud's is without an underlying disease or associated medical problem that could provoke vasospasm. Also called Raynaud's disease, it's the most common form of the disorder. Primary Raynaud's typically affects the digits of both hands and both feet. Secondary Raynaud's. This is Raynaud's caused by an underlying problem. Also called Raynaud's phenomenon, secondary Raynaud's usually affects both of your hands or both feet. Although secondary Raynaud's is less common than the primary form, it's often a more complex and serious disorder.

Causes of Secondary Raynaud's

- **Scleroderma.** Raynaud's phenomenon occurs in the majority of people who have scleroderma, a rare disease that leads to hardening and scarring of the skin. Scleroderma, a type of connective tissue disease, results in Raynaud's disease because it reduces blood flow to the extremities. It causes tiny blood vessels in the hands and feet to thicken and to constrict too easily, promoting Raynaud's.

- **Lupus erythematousus.** Raynaud's is also a common problem for people with lupus—an "autoimmune" disease (as viewed by conventional medicine) that can affect many parts of your body, including your skin, joints, organs, and blood vessels. An autoimmune disease is one in which your immune system attacks healthy tissue, (conventional viewpoint).

- **Rheumatoid arthritis.** Raynaud's may be an initial sign of rheumatoid arthritis, an inflammatory condition causing pain and stiffness in the joints, often including the hands and feet.

- **Sjogren's syndrome.** Raynaud's phenomenon can also occur in people who have Sjogren's syndrome — a rare disorder that often accompanies scleroderma, lupus or rheumatoid arthritis. The hallmark of Sjogren's syndrome, a connective tissue disease, is chronic dryness of the eyes and mouth.

- **Diseases of the arteries.** Raynaud's phenomenon can be associated with various diseases that affect the arteries, such as atherosclerosis, which is the gradual buildup of plaque in the blood vessels that feed the heart (coronary arteries), or Buerger's disease, a disorder in which the blood vessels of the hands and feet become inflamed. Primary pulmonary hypertension, a type of high blood pressure that affects only the arteries of the lungs, is frequently associated with Raynaud's.

- **Carpal tunnel syndrome.** The carpal tunnel is a narrow passageway in your wrist that protects a major nerve to your hand. Carpal tunnel syndrome is a condition in which pressure is put on this nerve, producing numbness and pain in the affected hand. The affected hand may become more susceptible to cold temperatures and episodes of Raynaud's."

- **Repetitive trauma.** Raynaud's can also be caused by repetitive trauma that damages nerves serving blood vessels in the hands and feet. In fact, nerve damage is thought to play a role in many cases of Raynaud's. Some people who type or play the piano vigorously or for long periods of time may be susceptible to Raynaud's. Workers who operate vibrating tools can develop a type of Raynaud's phenomenon called vibration-induced white finger.

- **Smoking.** Smoking constricts blood vessels and is a potential cause of Raynaud's.

- **Injuries.** Prior injuries to the hands or feet, such as a wrist fracture, surgery, or frostbite, can lead to Raynaud's phenomenon.

- **Certain medications**. The following drugs have been linked to Raynaud's phenomenon: Beta blockers, which are used to treat high blood pressure; migraine headache medications that contain ergotamine; medications containing estrogen; certain chemotherapy agents; and drugs that cause blood vessels to narrow, such as some over-the-counter cold medications.

- **Chemical exposure**. Some workers in the plastics industry who are exposed to vinyl chloride develop an illness similar to scleroderma. Raynaud's can be a part of that illness.

- **Other causes.** Raynaud's has also been linked to an underactive thyroid gland (hypothyroidism) and, rarely, to certain cancers."

Systemic Lupus Erythematosus Reversed

Systemic lupus erythematosus (SLE) is a chronic disease that causes inflammation in connective tissues, which provide strength and flexibility to structures throughout the body;these include cartilage and the lining of blood vessels. The signs and symptoms of SLE vary among affected individuals, and can involve many organs and systems, including the skin, joints, kidneys, lungs, central nervous system, and blood-forming (hematopoietic) system. SLE is one of a large group of conditions the medical community calls "autoimmune" disorders that occur when the immune system attacks the body's own tissues and organs.

As described above, systemic lupus erythematosus is yet another falsely labeled "autoimmune" disease. In 2016, I had a family fly in from Iowa for treatment. The grandmother had been diagnosed by a medical doctor with SLE, and the daughter, who was 42 at the time, was diagnosed with right kidney dysfunction, which she had had since the age of five.

During my initial examination, I asked the grandmother if she had taken any medications during her pregnancy. She replied yes, she was given a prescription, Bendectin, for nausea. Bendectin is similar to thalidomide, which caused irreparable damage to many children by causing flipper malformations of the hands. When I examined the grandmother, she still had remnants of the Bendectin trapped in her liver. Since she was pregnant with her daughter at the time she took the medication, I tested the daughter and found the Bendectin trapped in the daughter's right kidney. The question arises, how do we get these nasty drugs out of the body? The answer is simple:, with a homeopathic nosode, that is, a homeopathic dilution of the actual drug. Because there were so many lawsuits, Bendectin was taken off the market in 1985. I could not locate it anywhere in the United States. I called my good friend, Peter, in Canada and fortunately he was able to locate the drug at his compounding pharmacy. After getting samples of the drug, I made homeopathic dilutions. The grandmother required a 30C potency and the daughter needed a 200C potency. In six weeks after treating the daughter with the homeopathic remedy, her right kidney problem totally resolved. It took nine months of treatment for the mother's "autoimmune" disease, lupus to disappear. Do you still believe in the fairy tale that the body attacks itself for no apparent reason?

Another Autoimmune Fairy Tale:
Dental-Rheumatoid Arthritis Connection

M.T. was a 64-year-old Caucasian female who worked as a medical transcriptionist. In 1974, a diagnosis of rheumatoid arthritis (RA) was made. At the early age of 30, she presented clinical symptoms of swollen knees. Through the years, her condition gradually worsened until she experienced severe painful joints throughout her body. M.T.'s medical treatment included the use of the steroid, prednisone, a chemotherapy drug, methotrexate, and a deactivating drug, Enbrel. The yearly cost for just the Enbrel alone was $13,500, which was paid for by her insurance company.

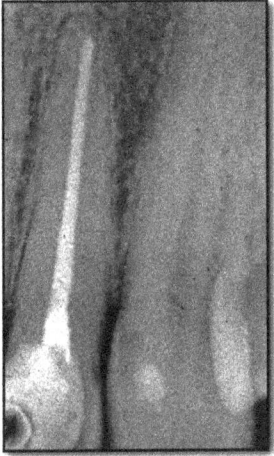

X-Rays Don't Show Infections in Dentinal Tubules.

Rheumatoid arthritis affects millions of Americans. It is considered a chronic joint disease that causes the soft tissue around the joints to thicken and swell and cartilage to erode. Unlike osteoarthritis, which is characterized by joint damage from wear-and-tear stress, RA is a disease in which the body's own immune system attacks the joints, especially the joints of the hands and feet. It is for this reason that RA is thought to be an "autoimmune disease."

Enbrel is primarily used to block the tumor necrosis factor alpha (TNF alpha), which the body produces during the inflammatory response, that is, the body's reaction to injury. TNF alpha promotes the inflammation and its associated fever and signs (pain, tenderness, and swelling) in several inflammatory conditions, including RA. From a healing perspective, inflammation is the first step in the body's attempt to heal. Whether bacterial, viral, fungal, or chemical substances concentrate in an area, the body must react to remove the offending agent(s). From a clinical perspective, it is totally illogical for the body to initiate a process that would attack itself for no good reason. In fact, most "autoimmune" diseases have an underlying factor ("splinter"), that traditional medicine has not yet been able to recognize.

One overlooked source for initiating RA are dental foci. Dental infections, whether from an infected root canal tooth, gum disease, or sites of previously extracted teeth (cavitations), all provide the potential of 300 to 400 different pathogens. Bacteria, viruses, and fungi or any combination plus degenerating protein substances from tooth structures produce toxins (thiolethers, hydrogen sulfide, and mercaptans) which circulate throughout the entire body. Concentration of poisonous substances within a knee, hand, finger, or other joint will cause inflammation. This was true in M.T.'s case. Within one to two years before the onset of her RA, she had a root canal treatment performed on an upper left lateral incisor. This seemingly innocuous dental procedure resulted in a Streptococcus inflection that remained in her body for 34 years. An x-ray of the treated tooth showed no visible pathology. Unfortunately, a high percentage of root canal treated teeth (75% or more) become infected. Although they exhibit none of the usual clinical signs and symptoms of pain, swelling, or redness, they can spew out their toxic waste products that affect distant sites.

A noninvasive approach utilizing technology developed in the 1930's was used to resolve the *streptococcal* infection within the tooth. Following two treatment sessions, M.T.'s RA resolved by 90%, and she stopped taking the Enbrel. No additional therapy was instituted at the time of treatment. This patient has regained a pain-free quality of life. The key factor was the removal of the underlying cause -- a *Streptococcal* infection within the root canal tooth -- which started the release of the TNF.

Use of medications to block TNF or any other components of the inflammatory process only treats the symptoms NOT the actual cause. The belief in an "autoimmune" component of the disease process is often adhered to because physicians do not understand the nature of the dental component in the disease process.

Dental-Congestive Heart Failure Connection

Another cure that has eluded the medical establishment is for congestive heart failure. As mentioned earlier, the physician must diagnose the root cause instead of treating the symptoms.

Idiopathic Cardiomyopathy

When the cause of heart failure is never identified, it is referred to as idiopathic cardiomyopathy. This condition can be caused by past-unidentified viral or bacterial infections. Unfortunately, most cardiologists do not investigate the possibility that existing dental infections can play a major role in causing congestive heart failure. According to Dr. Dietrich Klinghardt, M.D., Ph.D., 70% of all medical problems have their origin in the mouth. From my own clinical experience over the past thirty-seven years, I believe this estimate may even be conservative. One of the primary reasons the dental component of the disease process is ignored is because in most instances the patient does not have any complaints about his or her mouth. Most infections in the mouth that provide a focus for causing distant medical problems do not manifest any swelling or painful conditions. Most scenarios involve an old root canal tooth or postextraction site that harbors viruses or bacteria whose toxins disseminate throughout the body and concentrate in a particular organ, such as the heart, causing dysfunction for which physicians cannot find a cause. Approximately 90% of postextraction sites (mostly wisdom teeth but other sites can be involved) have a residual infection remaining in the jawbone that does NOT show up on regular dental x-rays. In my opinion, the major causes for this frequent occurrence are due to failure to achieve primary closure of the soft tissue (gum) with sutures after tooth removal; failure to "sterilize" the extraction site with ozone; failure to remove infected bone that lines the socket; and failure to remove infected root remnants in the jaw bone resulting from root tip fractures. If the surgeon is unable to accomplish primary closure, he or she must protect the wound by placing and suturing in a resorbable sponge

(Gelfoam) saturated with homeopathic remedies in the socket. This then reduces pathogens and debris from entering the socket during the healing process.

Mrs. Jung's husband, who is a practicing dentist in Seoul, Korea, brought his wife to our office in Langhorne, Pennsylvania. Mrs. Jung, who was in her early 40's, had been suffering from congestive heart failure (CHF) for ten years. Despite the fact that she was examined and diagnosed with CHF by leading cardiologists in Korea, her condition did not respond to medications and her cardiologists were unable to uncover the source of her problem. Examination by direct resonance testing revealed the presence of a *streptococcal* infection in the lower right jawbone area where a third molar had been removed ten years before. Soon after the extraction, the CHF symptoms appeared. Mrs. Jung's primary symptoms included severe fatigue, memory loss and mental fog, shortness of breath, and leg edema. Other CHF patients exhibit additional symptoms, as noted below.

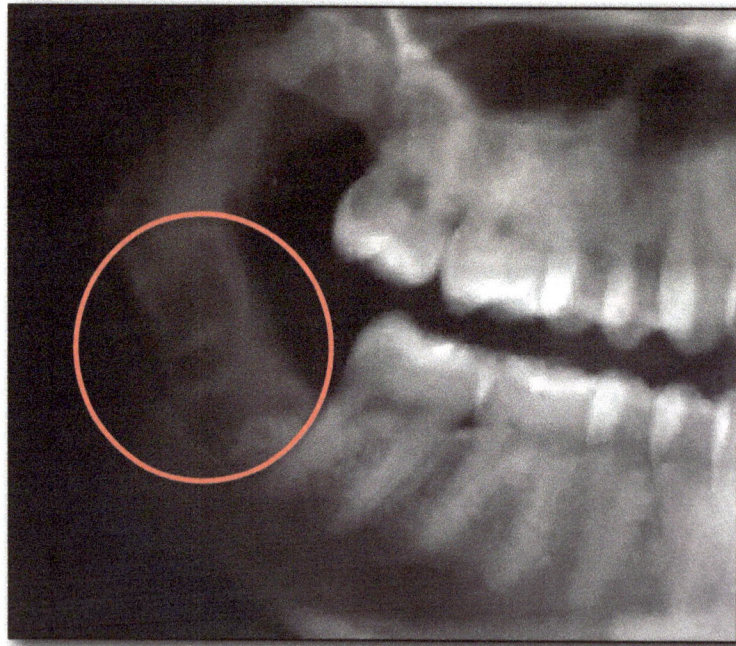

Symptoms of heart failure vary and include the following

Fatigue	Nausea
Increased heart rate, palpitations	Persistent coughing or wheezing
Loss of appetite	Shortness of breath (dyspnea)
Memory loss, confusion	Swelling (edema) of the feet, legs, or abdomen

The toxins produced by the residual *streptococcal* infection are capable of entering the thyroid, thereby weakening the heart muscle so that it is unable to adequately pump blood throughout the body and/or unable to prevent blood from "backing up" into the lungs. In most cases, this process occurs over time, when an underlying condition damages the heart or makes it work too hard, weakening the organ.

Once the underlying pathogen, *streptococcus*, was diagnosed, appropriate nutritional support was given to enhance the body's immune system. Within six to eight weeks, Mrs. Jung's CHF symptoms of ten-years' duration totally resolved.

The red circled area on the x-ray above depicts the post-surgical third molar extraction site. There appears to be a cavitation, which is the area of infection. Energetic testing diagnosed the *streptococcus* infection.

Congestive Heart Failure / Dental Connection

It's more common than you would believe. Virginia Coomer was a 77-year-old female who was diagnosed with CHF and had been treated with the drug digoxin for the past ten years. When Virginia was first referred to my office, she could hardly walk to the treatment room. When she finally did make it into the room, she was huffing and puffing and out of breath. During the ten-year period that Virginia was on the

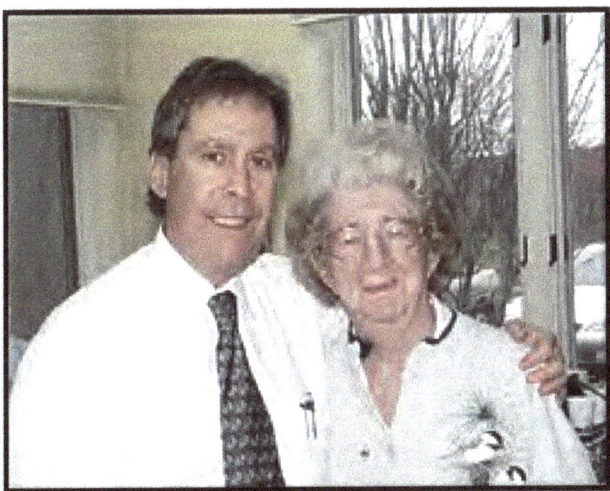

heart medication, her condition deteriorated to the point where she could not live a normal life. She basically was home bound because she did not have the strength to do anything.

A clinical evaluation revealed that Virginia had a major dental problem that was contributing to her distress level. A full upper and lower partial denture was fabricated in 1968. Even the best constructed denture must be replaced in eight to ten years. Virginia's dentures were thirty-four-years-old. A lot of major changes had taken place, such as wearing down of the denture teeth and shrinking of the supporting bone. These alterations resulted in the shifting of skull bones, compression of the spine, and rotation of the pelvis. Another major complaint that Virginia had, was severe groin pain that had defied medical diagnosis for the past three years. The ill-fitting dentures played a significant role in distressing (Dental Distress Syndrome) the nervous and musculoskeletal systems. It is statistically known that patients with dentures are among the most medically compromised group of patients and have the highest rate of chronic illnesses.

By means of direct resonance testing, Virginia was shown to have an underactive thyroid even though she was taking the thyroid medication, Synthroid. Testing also revealed that her heart responded well to specific nutrients known to support repair of heart tissue (protomorphogens, antioxidants, amino acids, vitamins, and minerals). Each supplement MUST be tested for compatibility with the patient's system in order to provide maximum effectiveness. Shotgunning patients with a "standardized" protocol of nutrients is inappropriate treatment, since every patient is a chemical and energetic individual. After testing, five nutrients where shown to match and support the patient's nutritional needs. The incredible result was that Virginia responded to treatment in just one week. At her second visit, she walked into the treatment room effortlessly with NO huffing and puffing and more energy than she had had in ten years. When Virginia's husband called their family physician to tell him that Virginia's CHF was reversed, he replied, "the medication finally kicked in (after ten years)." I am convinced that some physicians take a course in medical school called BS 101.

In six weeks, Virginia's life was restored to normal activities. She now has a new lease on life and eagerly engages in as much activity as her husband's physical stamina will allow. In addition, after restoring the integrity of her dentures (cranial bone adjustment, relining the upper and lower dentures, and restoring vertical jaw height), her groin pain of three-years duration resolved by 98 percent. The head bone is connected to the neck bone and the neck bone is connected to the pelvis.

The nutritional component of congestive heart disease has not been well understood by most physicians. Traditional attention has focused on nutrients such as the antioxidants: beta-carotene (vitamin A), vitamin C, vitamin E, and selenium, three of the B-vitamins: vitamin B-6, vitamin B-12, and folic acid, calcium, magnesium, and coenzyme Q10. Although these nutrients are essential, there are more effective ones that will specifically support heart muscle function and repair. The proof is seen in another CHF case report of Walter Kruse, whose medical records documented that repair of the mitral value and right ventricle occurred in seven months with just natural vitamin supplements. The technology to reverse congestive heart failure is available. One just has to make the correct choices and find the right physician.

Reversing Congestive Heart Failure

Of all newly diagnosed patients, 50% of heart failure patients die within 5 years of diagnosis. This is a frightening statistic and one that drives home the fact that traditional medicine treats only symptoms. In traditional medical literature it states, "In the majority of cases, it results from an underlying disease, such as coronary artery disease or hypertension, which has damaged or weakened the heart. Thus, heart failure itself is not considered a disease, but rather a condition produced by a disease or diseases." There is NO mention of any NUTRITIONAL deficiencies as a major cause for CHF.

Doctor Royal Lee, a dentist, demonstrated in the 1930's that processed foods (white sugar, milled and bleached flour) was the direct cause of heart arrhythmias, faulty electrical conduction (heart block due to a deficiency of vitmain B-4 [only found in food-based nutrients]), and weakening of the heart muscle (hypothyroidism or tyrosine deficiency). He also proved that in many instances that the addition of specific natural food supplements would result in immediate reversals of heart irregularities (e.g., extra heart sounds, rapid heartbeat, skipped beats). His research is as valid today as it was back in the 1930's.

A weakened heart has to work harder to pump the proper amount of blood. To compensate for the heavier workload, it may beat faster and enlarge. This compensatory mechanism can temporarily increase pumping capacity but will eventually accelerate the progression of heart failure. When heart function becomes dramatically reduced, patients are often winded and fatigued by exertion, sometimes making even the task of tying one's shoes difficult. If the heart further loses its ability to pump blood to the vital organs, heart failure can be fatal. The following are the more common symptoms observed by patients:

Shortness of breath (dyspnea). This is one of the earliest symptoms of heart failure. The patient gets winded and fatigued more quickly than before, just by doing regular daily activities or even lying in bed. There is also decreased tolerance to exercise, and the muscles may feel weaker than before.

Swelling (edema) of the legs is another common symptom in heart failure, though it could also be caused by unrelated conditions.

Swollen neck veins.

Abdominal discomfort such as swelling, pain or nausea.

Mental confusion.

Galloping heartbeat (palpitations).

Kidney malfunction or failure (in the later stages of CHF).

What physicians call heart disease is really caused by nutritional deficiencies and adulterated omega-6 oils. Unless stipulated on the label, as "organic and cold pressed," most oils are processed to extend their shelf-life. When these corrupted omega-6 oils enter the body and get integrated into the bloodless cell membranes throughout the body, they cause inflammation. It is the inflammation that provides the basis for fibrosis (scarring) of the cell membrane and decreased oxygen levels in the cell. When the oxygen level drops by 35% continuously, then cancer, diabetes, and cardiomyopathy develop. It's not a disease it's adulterated foods that are causing our illnesses.

In addition to the symptoms listed above, which the patient may notice, the physician may also be able to detect signs of CHF, which include the following:

An abnormal heart murmur (a telltale sign of a valve-related disorder).

A crackling sound of fluid in the lungs (rales), which is a sign of pulmonary congestion.

A rapid heartbeat (tachycardia) or irregular heart rhythms (arrhythmias).

Swelling and fluid retention (edema) in the liver or gastrointestinal tract (in advanced stages of CHF).

Hypertrophy or enlargement of the heart.

Liver malfunction.

Emphysema: Dental Connection

Robert had suffered from emphysema for many years. He was placed on steroids for the past year and a half. Fortunately, Robert worked with one of our patients who referred him to my office. A comprehensive examination revealed a *strepococcal* infection in the upper jaw bone where a second bicuspid tooth had been removed ten years previously. Once the *strepococcal* infection was resolved without drugs, Robert's emphysema disappeared.

The cases presented in this book and those listed on my website: www.icnr.com, all have a common theme: find the "splinters" and remove them and watch the body heal. The answers to the patients' medical problems are readily accessible if you ask the right questions and know what to look for. Finding the solution is easier than you think.

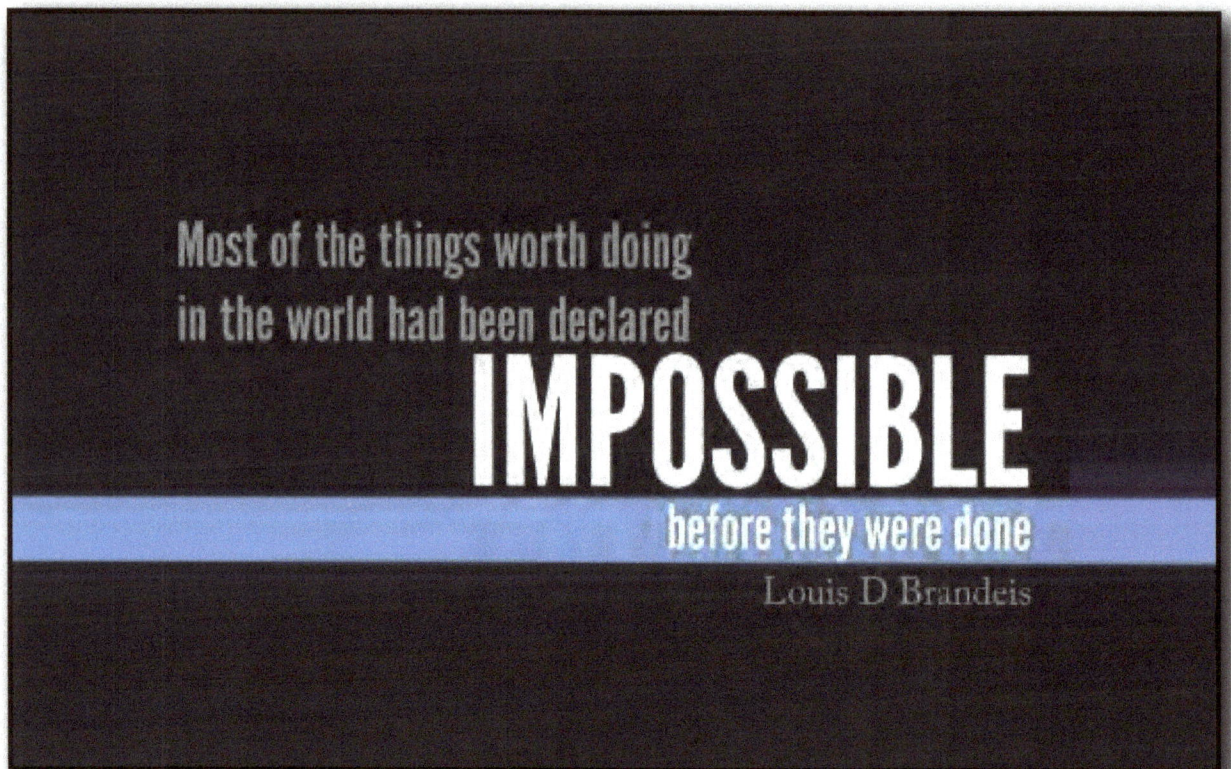

Most of the things worth doing in the world had been declared **IMPOSSIBLE** before they were done

Louis D Brandeis

Psychological Complex

The mind is the most powerful healing mechanism we have. It can also be the most destructive mechanism humans have. If a patient goes into an oncologist, and the doctor tells the patient you only have two months to live, and the patient buys into the prognosis, he or she invariably dies exactly in two months. The mind has the ability to shut down its immune system and program the body to self-destruction. In reality, it is the mind that dictates the physiology of the cells. This concept is called epigenetics: the study of changes in organisms caused by modification of gene expression rather than alteration of the genetic code itself. In plain language, what it means is that your environment really dictates how the cells react. If you operate in fear mode, your system will deteriorate rapidly. If you fake it until you make it, your body will respond positively. A perfect example follows. While cycling for the American Cancer Society, I met a retired motor cycle policemen. Nick was diagnosed with colon cancer twenty-two years before I met him. He refused traditional medical treatment. He told me he went to church every morning and prayed. He also told me he changed his diet 180 degrees. In six months, his cancer disappeared. Mind over matter. YES! Your thought process dictates how your cells function. Putting in some Sunoco racing fuel (good organic vegetables) doesn't hurt either.

As Dr. Bruce Lipton, the cellular biologist, has stated many times in his interviews, the mind is preprogramed before the age of seven. We are like computer hard drives. Our ancestral genetics (software codes) are transferred to us at the time of gestation (union of the egg and the sperm). Our behavioral patterns are learned from our immediate environment. Like a duckling imprinting on its mother. We visually and auditorially record behavioral patterns and learn the rules of life. If you were fortunate enough to grow up in a nurturing environment and exposed to an abundance of positive attitudes, then you are well equipped to handle the journey. If the opposite applies, then the probability exists that you will have a bumpy journey through life and may not even realize where it all came from.

In 1936, Hans Selye, M.D., the "Father" of Stress and Distress, showed experimentally that the adrenal glands ("fight or flight" mechanism) react the same way to physical, chemical, or psychological distress. The body cannot differentiate among the three stressors. When the adrenals get stimulated, they release over sixty different hormones and they all need cholesterol to be produced. One of the primary hormones they produce is cortisol. Cortisol is a catabolic hormone that tears down your body. This is why meditation, exercise, Pilates, and yoga are so important. They destress the body. Those who live a stressful life will age more quickly because of the effects of cortisol. No matter what healing approach you embark on to restore your health, you must also take command of your emotions if you want to succeed in achieving a high level of health.

In 1988, I studied with a chiropractor, Dr. Scot Walker, from Encinitas California, who was teaching NET, Neuro Emotional Technique. NET is useful to help process and release stress-related issues — both in mind and body. It also is capable of releasing reflex physiological and structural responses to the mental stressors. During Dr. Walkers' workshop, we practiced on each other to learn the technique. I was plagued by an upper left trapezius trigger point that I could not get rid of. My training partner tracked it down to an emotional issue I had with one of my wife's best friends who like a first sergeant in the army always trying to control everything. Personally, I found her very annoying but endured the relationship because of my wife. Following the tapping procedure to erase my body's reflex action to my mental image of her, my trigger point totally disappeared and has never returned. I have used this technique on many of my patients through the years with great results.

In another example, one of my patient's best friend passed away, and she became emotionally very distraught over the death. The key to erasing the response to the emotional trauma is to perform a kinesilogic test to find which organ(s) is the weak link. Each organ relates to a specific set of emotions which are related to each emotional event that affects the patient. By tapping the vertebrae that neurologically connect to the pre-tested weak organs and emotions, the body's reflex response to that incident can be totally erased while the patient thinks about the emotional issue. The tapping on the spine disrupts and eliminates the physiologic response related to the emotion attached to the event. The mental event cannot be changed; however, the body's response to it can be removed. NET is a great technique to help patients overcome adversity.

Often patients do not realize that their pain and/or dysfunction is emotionally related. One of my patients, Rose, had severe chronic migraine headaches. For a year and a half I tried all different techniques but nothing worked. Three years after the patient left my practice, I received a call from Rose. She informed me that her migraines headaches were completely gone. When I asked her what she did to get rid of her migraines, she replied she did nothing. When I asked her what had changed, she said "Lou died." She stated that as soon as her husband died, her migraines disappeared. From that moment on, I became a big believer in psychosomatic pain.

Real Cause of Alzheimer's and Dementia

Worldwide, 50 million people are living with Alzheimer's and other dementias. Alzheimer's disease is a degenerative brain disease and the most common form of dementia. Dementia is not a specific disease.

Scientists believe the problem begins with the slow degeneration of the brain cells by two abnormal structures: plaques and tangles. It is thought that the plaques and tangles are the prime cause for damaging and killing nerve cells. The plaque consists of deposits of beta-amyloid, which is a protein fragment that builds up in the spaces between the nerve cells.

The tangles on the other hand are twisted fibers of another protein called tau that build up within the cells. Most experts believe both the plaque and tangles play a critical role in blocking communication among the cells and disrupting the normal cell's processes.

Based on my fifty years of clinical experience, I have concluded that the presence of the plaque and tangles is based on a reaction to an alteration within in the brain tissue. The potential factors that can elicit such changes can be derived from three sources: physical, chemical, and psychological. Structural distortions such as a concussion, which will alter the blood flow and accumulate metabolic wastes and initiate inflammation, scarring, and degeneration can potentially be the cause for build-up of plaque and tangles.

A second group of causes include chemicals and heavy metal toxicity from root canal teeth (methyl mercaptans, hydrogen sulfide, and thioethers), mercury fillings, arsenic laden pesticides used on chicken feed, chemtrail contaminants (aluminum, barium, and strontium), radiation from Fukushima, Japan (March 2011), the herbicide glyphosate (Monsanto's Round-Up), viruses like cytomegalovirus, Epstein-Barr virus, Lyme infection, and a myriad of other environmental chemicals. Another important aspect is the fact that most peoples' membranes are inflamed from the adulterated fats in our food, especially the omega-6 fatty acids (corn, canola, safflower, sunflower, and soy). Once corrupted by the adulterated oils, the amount of oxygen entering the cell is dramatically reduced. A perfect storm in the form of Alzheimer's disease is just a matter of time.

The third factor is psychological. Dr. Ryke Geerd Hamer, originator of the New German Medicine, has shown that emotional traumas can form calcium deposits in the brain and ultimately form cancer anywhere in the body. The common denominator of all three groups is that they will initiate inflammation. Chronic inflammation will result in fibrosis or scaring, which in turn will cause decrease circulation, a build-up of toxic wastes, and ultimately cellular dysfunction.

In my professional opinion, the plaque and tangles are a direct reaction of the body to the chronic inflammation and its sequela. Depending on where the degeneration occurs in the brain, the location will dictate the symptomatology exhibited by the patient.

A recent case provided validation of my theory.

Case Study: Alzheimer's

Patrick Loftus was referred to me for evaluation of moderate to severe Alzheimer's symptoms. When Patrick first came for evaluation, he had a glazed look on his face like a deer caught in headlights. He also was unable to follow instructions and physically had to be put into the examining chair. Employing Quantum Testing Techniques, I diagnosed glyphosate, Lyme, and mercury on the left side of his brain. A nutritional program was tested to select specific nutrients to remove the offending "splinters" present. A comprehensive program was also established to prepare his body for the detoxification process. After three months of treatments, Patrick was fully cognizant and was able to follow directions. Unfortunately, his speech was not fully understandable, but he made a concerted effort to express his thoughts. Of interest, the mercury that was diagnosed in his brain was located in the Broca speech center. Do you think there is a correlation?

Patrick's wife, Lauren, is a certified conventionally trained nurse and was amazed at the progress her husband made in just three months. The medications that Patrick was prescribed were primarily to control his symptoms, but he showed no significant improvement.

None of the physicians had any idea of what was in his brain even possible contaminants. In

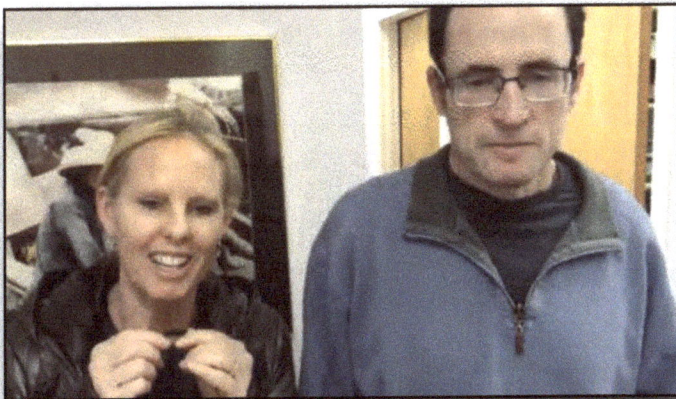

View Video at www.icnr.com/splvideo/

additions, Lauren had to leave Patrick with his parents while she arranged a move to Sarasota, Florida. His parents were also truly amazed at their son's progress is such a short time. I believe that with further treatment using specific nutrients for brain repair and scalar energy that Patrick will gain more skills and improved speech.

A Powerful New Way to Edit DNA

Russian scientific research directly or indirectly explains phenomena such as clairvoyance, intuition, spontaneous and remote acts of healing, self-healing, affirmation techniques, unusual light/auras around people (namely spiritual masters), the mind's influence on weather patterns, and much more. In addition, there is evidence for a whole new type of medicine in which DNA can be influenced and reprogrammed by words and frequencies WITHOUT cutting out and replacing single genes.

Frequencies For Healing the Brain

In the 1960s, researchers were using frequencies to resolve alcohol and heroin addiction in three to five days. The primary reason it never was accepted is that it would have destroyed an entire rehabilitation industry.

For those who have access to biofrequency devices like the Rife generator, they can conveniently treat themselves. One can easily restore calmness and erase feelings of dependency by running a frequency sweep from 111 Hertz to 112 Hertz for 30 minutes per day for 5 days. The frequency range will stimulate all the neurotransmitters and re-establish a sense of well-being. The frequency chart below is provided to assist in helping your body heal.

From a nutritional perspective, one needs to take several supplements to restore brain function: organic cold pressed omega-6, omega-3, and gama linolenic fatty acids. This special proprietary blend is unadulterated, organic and cold pressed. The toxic overload that we get from the adulterated omega-6 oils (corn, soy, safflower, sunflower, grape seed, and canola) that is in our everyday food supply is corrupting our cell membranes. **It is the adulterated omega-6 oils that are pro-inflammatory and not the organic, cold pressed form.** An adulterated cell membrane reduces oxygen flow into the cells. It also prevents the production of omega-3 derivatives like DHA (docosahexaenoic acid) and EPA (eicosapentaenoic acid), of which the brain only requires 7.2 mg per day. If your cardiologist recommended you take any form of fish oil, please stop immediately. All fish oils become rancid at room temperature and completely rancid in the body at 98.6^0 F. Also, it takes eighteen weeks to exit your body once you discontinue the oils.

Systemic Enzymes

One of the underlying causes of reduced brain function is fibrosis or scaring of the brain tissue. Once irritants such as chemicals, pesticides, herbicides, heavy metals, viruses, bacteria, vaccines and their adjuvants enter the brain, they cause inflammation. It is the constant inflammation that causes the scarring. The best way to reverse the fibrosis is to take a systemic enzyme. The best one available and the most clinically successful is the product, Zymessence available from WAM Essentials, Inc. (1-866-268-3216); it literally digests the excess fibrin (scars) in the brain, and everywhere else in the body, increases circulation in the micro-capillary system, and reduces your chances of getting dementia.

Adaptogens

The last essential supplement is cordyceps. The fungus must be grown at high altitudes (above 3000 meters or 10,000 feet) in a pristine environment with the correct moisture levels. Most cordyceps sold in the United States comes from either the U.S. or Canada. These products are not potent enough. Cordyceps increases ATP (adenosine triphosphate) in the mitochondria, which is the primary ingredient for energy production. It also stimulates and directs stem cells to form whatever cells are needed for repair and is a modulator in the body. It is an adaptogenic substance, that is, it enables organs to recuperate quicker and helps bring overworked and under functioning organs back to homeostasis or balance.

Biofrequencies

In the 1930s, Raymond Royal Rife invented a microscope, with a magnification five times more powerful than the traditional light microscopes that were being used in the university research centers. Dr. Rife was viewing viruses and other pathogens that traditional researchers did not know existed. From his innovative universal microscope, he was able to determine the mortal oscillatory frequency at which pathogens vibrated. Dr. Rife then partnered with Lee de Forest, the inventor of the vacuum tube, to construct a functional generator. This device was capable of producing frequencies that could destroy disease causing bacteria and viruses. Dr. Rife was successful in curing many diseases at that time and even curing cancer. For the incredible story about Dr. Rife, his microscope, and the cure for cancer, I recommend you read the book, *The Cancer Cure That Worked: Fifty Years of Suppression* by Barry Lynes.

In addition to curing various diseases, the Rife frequency generator was used to treat many other problems that plagued patients such as pain, hormone imbalances, depression, addictions, insomnia, indigestion, to stimulate healing, and much more. The chart below provides special frequencies that have been effective in resolving numerous health issues. Many are aimed at reversing psychological issues for which traditional physicians use drugs.

Rife Healing Frequencies

432 Hertz	Transmits beneficial healing energies because it is a pure tone of mathematics fundamental to nature.
444 Hertz	Kills cancer cells.
174 Hertz	Pain relief
Sweep 90 Hertz to 111 Hertz	Release beta endorphins for pain relief
197 Hertz	Restores love of others, warmth (1 hour session)
528 Hertz	Repair DNA. Brings Positive Transformation

432 Hertz	Transmits beneficial healing energies because it is a pure tone of mathematics fundamental to nature.
417 Hertz	Wipes out all the Negative Energy
10,000 Hertz	Regeneration Regrowth Repair Frequencies; All 7 Chakras; 12 Meridians Chi Energy
456 Hertz	Head cold, Sinus infection
852 Hertz	LET Go of Fear, Overthinking & Worries / Cleanse Destructive Energy / Awakening Intuition
5 Hz, 26 Hz, 79 Hz, 80 Hz, 82 Hz	For pain.
7 Hz, 70 Hz, 85 Hz	Acute pain.
76 Hertz	Chronic pain
11 Hz, 17 Hz, 53 Hz, 55 Hz, and 71 Hz	Emotional issues
7 Hz, 66 Hz	Rheumatoid Arthritis.
7.83 Hertz	Schumann Resonance (frequency of the earth)
1465 Hertz	Reestablished a sense of well-being

Remember that a two minute cell phone call stimulates the alpha, beta, delta, and theta brain waves and requires 2 hours for the brain to settle down.

A Powerful Exercise for Initiating DNA Repair and Cellular Rejuvenation

The use of guided visualization and imagery is growing in acceptance as a complementary healing modality, particularly in stress reduction, and easing pain, suffering, and other consequences of cancer and its treatment. Significant data indicate that the emotional trauma associated with a cancer diagnosis and the side effects of treatment can be minimized in some people who practice imagery. An important concept to know is that the immune cells are not the primary removers of "toxic" cells. Your imagery must focus on a DNA spiral model for fixing genetic errors. By placing your hands in a tent formation and placing them over your navel area (major acupuncture point, conception vessel), you begin visualizing the toxic substances (heavy metals, pesticides, viruses, chemicals, cancer cells, etc.) leaving your body, and then visualize energy coming into your body to enhance DNA repair and cellular rejuvenation. When you place your hands over the navel area you will sense the increased energy flow. Meditate for fifteen minutes upon awakening to energize your body before you start the day.

This process can be enhanced by using a technique developed by Dr. Stanley Ngui* called the Qigong Matrix System. Tap with your nail from your middle finger in a figure "8" pattern over your eyebrows, across the bridge of the nose and repeat in a horizontal figure "8" around both eyes for fifteen minutes. This relaxes the brain and energizes the entire body. The Qigong Matrix System is based on 23 generations of Qigong masters that have passed down this powerful art of healing. Correcting the energy flow enables the body to heal. Remember that drugs do not heal they only mask symptoms.

"Qi is that intangible energy that animates the human
body and all things in this Universe. "
~Richard Lee

"Qigong is a way of being.
Being soft, yet strong.
Qigong is a way of breathing.
Breathing deeply, yet calmly.
Qigong is a way of standing."
Alert, yet relaxed.
~Nigel Mills

* For those patients who continue to suffer pain and other ailments that traditional medicine has no answers, I strongly suggest contacting Nguistyle Integrative Medicine Clinic in Richmond Hill, Ontario (905.597.5007).

Chapter Nine - The Secret of Life, Longevity, and Anti-Aging

The Secret of Life, Longevity, and Reversing the Disease Process

Out of chaos comes stability. The common denominator of the universe and of life is scalar energy. Scalar energy exists in a longitudinal wave form capable of penetrating any solid object including Faraday Cages; it's capable of passing through the earth from one side to another with no loss of field strength (as proved in one of Nikola Tesla's research projects); it can travel billions of times faster than the speed of light (contrary to what Albert Einstein stated), and according to the Russian astrophysicist, Nikolai Kozyrev, scalar energy was the primal force for the creation of matter in the universe.

Scalar energy is recognized as a phase-conjugated double helix waveform that provides the template for repairing our DNA. Scalar energy also has the ability to disassemble toxins (heavy metals, chemicals, viruses, bacteria, and foreign substances) by altering their molecular structure, making them inert and non-reactive. Scalar energy also stimulates stems cells for repair. In essence, scalar energy is the "Holy Grail."

Exposing our bodies to full sunlight or using the Bioptron System of full spectrum light or the Theraphi System (actual scalar energy), eating raw organic food, meditating, prayer, and expressing positive affirmations all increase the body's scalar energy, which maintains our vitality.

Scalar energy supplies the power for cells to vibrate at their "factory default" frequency settings:

Brain frequencies average between 70-78 Hertz.	Liver: 55-60 Hz.
Thyroid and Parathyroid: 62-68 Hz.	Stomach: 58-65 Hz.
Thymus: 65-68 Hz.	Pancreas: 60-80 Hz.
Heart: 67-70 Hz.	Descending Colon: 58-63 Hz.
Lungs: 58-65 Hz.	Ascending Colon: 50-60 Hz.

Chapter Nine - The Secret of Life, Longevity, and Anti-Aging

Research has discovered that the general human healthy frequency of our body falls within the range of 62 to 72 Hz. When our bodies are assaulted by heavy metals, pesticides like glyphosate (Round–Up), vaccines, viruses, contaminated water, air, and processed foods (white sugar, white bread and white rice, etc.), chemtrails, toxic root canal teeth, genetically modified wheat, soy, corn, and other Frankenfoods from Monsanto, wi-fi and other EMFs, the body's frequency is lowered. When our frequency dips to 58 Hz we are more susceptible to colds and flu. When our frequency dips to 55 Hz we get colds and flu. When our frequency plummets to 42 Hz we get cancer. The prescription for anti-aging, prolonging our life, and reversing the disease process is simple. We must focus on reducing our exposure, as much as possible, to the aforementioned stressors plus putting Sunoco racing fuel (raw and unprocessed foods) into our bodies.

From a medical perspective, when we get sick, practitioners must define the core issues. Only through the use of vibrational technology (CyberScan, Direct Resonance or other energy based testing) can physicians detect the initiating factors. Once diagnosed and the initiators removed, the cells, tissues and organs can revert back to their "Factory Default" settings. As a practitioner of over 50 years of clinical experience, I have frequently witnessed this phenomenon. It makes no difference if we are dealing with the common cold or cancer. Once the offending initiators are removed, health is restored. The common denominator for achieving optimum health and increasing one's longevity and reversing disease is removing the initiators, detoxing the body, and eating real food all of which will restore the cell's frequencies. I refer you to review some of the 150 case studies on my website, www.icnr.com, to validate this concept. Remember, your health is your best insurance policy.

"All the money in the world can't buy you back good health."

Reba McEntire

Chapter Nine - The Secret of Life, Longevity, and Anti-Aging

CyberScan
Intelligent Evolution Through the Use of
Proprietary Scalar Wave Technology

The CyberScan[‡] determines your present and past health condition based on the trends that are identified in the current state of the body's immune system. With a database of over 135,000 electromagnetic signatures of information the CyberScan System can predict and modify an individual's personal future health.

Benefits of Cyberscan:

Reduce stress and anxiety	Improved general health
Improve athletic performance	Reduce aging factors
Improve sleep and dream recall	Enhanced muscle mobility
Enhanced mental clarity	Reduce digestive disorders
Reduce depression	Enhance detoxification
Reduce addictions	

Cyberscan supports and balances the immune system to reduce stress that may be caused by:

Infections	Geopathic Stress
Fungi	Radioactive Elements
Toxic Chemicals	Psyche: Emotional or Mental
Pesticides-Herbicides-Insecticides	Energetic Distortions
Mercury and other Heavy Metals	Teeth
Electro-smog	

Ten-Second Scan

CyberScan quickly scans the morphogenetic or energy fields around cells, determines where the stressors are within the body, and creates a 100% natural scalar information carrier that communicates, as well as stimulates, the self-healing properties of the immune system.

eeCARD

CyberScan creates a personalized, electro-magnetic protection card designed specifically to protect your immune system from electro-smog and geopathic stress. When carried in your pocket, it protects you on a daily basis.

CyberScan Philosophy

During the past 25 years patients have witnessed incredible advances in medical technology which have improved their quality of life. As a result of this intelligent evolution, the CyberScan Professional System evolved. This system has incorporated the genius of Nicola Tesla's discovery of scalar waves and the most advanced concepts of Quantum Physics. The benefits of this integration is that health problems can now be solved more cost effectively. By using noninvasive scalar wave technology practitioners can now correct abnormal energy fields surrounding cells. When the morphogenic or energy field around the cell becomes normalized it communicates this information to the internal parts and reprograms the cell to work normally. When cells function normally the symptoms disappear.

CyberScan's Innovative Healing Process

The CyberScan System approaches health issues in several ways. First phase detects the underlying cause(s) of your problem. The detox process takes approximately three months. Most patients are seen every two weeks to be rescanned. If your health issues are more serious, you may require more attention on a weekly basis. CyberScan also addresses EMFs (Electromagnetic Frequencies), wi-fi, cell phone frequencies and much more. A custom eeCard is specifically programed to meet your needs. By placing this card under the foot of your bed it protects against potentially dangerous frequencies during sleep. This "insurance" policy helps you obtain a more restful nights sleep. In addition, the card can be worn during the day for continued protection.

Chapter Nine -The Secret of Life, Longevity, and Anti-Aging

Phase two focuses on regeneration during the second three month period. Once the offending factors are removed the scalar waves start the restoration of normal healthy function.

† Cyberscan is not a diagnostic tool. It is not intended to Diagnose, Treat, or Cure Disease or Illness, nor is it to be presented or construed, in any way, as a substitute for Professional Medical, Surgical or Psychiatric Care or Treatment.

‡ The CyberScan Professional System is a quantum physics based CE-Class IIa medical device in the EU and FDA registered as neurological biofeedback device. Made 100% in Germany. CyberScan utilizes state-of-the-art proprietary, scalar-energy technology based upon the patents and investigational trials of experimental physicist Nikola Tesla (1856-1943) and P.E.A.R. (Princeton Engineering Anomaly Research).

Theraphi Plasma System

In my 50 plus years of clinical practice, I have come to the conclusion that the common denominator for achieving real healing and health is with the use of scalar energy. The Theraphi Plasma System, which is now available in our practice, utilizes 18 specific healing frequencies coupled with a Bio-Active Plasma field of energy to affect cellular regeneration. When scalar energy and frequencies are combined their effect is much greater than either alone. A treatment session can vary between 6 and 18 minutes and is totally noninvasive. Repeat sessions can be safely accomplished with only a one hour hiatus.

An example of Theraphi's incredible effectiveness was recently witnessed when one of my patients who experienced left knee pain for five months had total resolution in two days with just two five minutes sessions. He had acupuncture, chiropractic and massage therapy during the five month period with no lasting results. Of interest, a decrease in the inflammatory process was documented by means of infrared photography. A dramatic decrease of 11.54^0F drop in temperature occurred immediately following treatment on the second day. The patient was in awe of the results.

The Theraphi Plasma System integrates the research of Royal Raymond Rife's healing frequencies from the 1930s, Nikola Tesla's noninvasive scalar wave electrotherapy from the 1920s, Antoine Priore's electromagnetic healing technology from the 1960s and '70s, and Georges Lakhovsky, a Russian physicist, while living in France, integrated the research of the three aforementioned pioneers. The ultimate benefit of the plasma generator is that the coherent electromagnetic field created by the Theraphi System restores your body to its original condition. In other words, your cells revert back to a "factory default" setting when every thing was in a state of health. This represents anti-aging at its finest.

The work of Vlail Kaznacheyev, a Russian researcher in the mid-1970s, showed that use of scalar electromagnetic waves can reverse cell death and the disease process. Rife, Priore, Lakhovsky, and Kaznacheyev successfully reversed cancers in both animals and humans.

By reversing the aging process this technology has been shown to be effective for:

• Pain reduction
• Reduction of inflammation
• Tissue regeneration
• Enhancing cancer remission
• Anti-aging
• Cell memory reversal

It becomes an obvious conclusion that if a cell that is in a pathologic, abnormal or diseased state can be reversed, then diseases such as MERSA (methicillin-resitant *Staphylococcus aureus*), Alzheimer's, dementia, heart disease, sports and other types of injuries and other medical illnesses can also be reversed.

Chapter Nine -The Secret of Life, Longevity, and Anti-Aging

In a "Cliff Notes" version, scalar energy enables practitioners to effectively heal pretty much any medical condition by correcting the mutated DNA.

Theraphi Plasma System

Why Is Scalar Energy So Effective?

The closer one gets to the truth the more simplistic the solution. Scalar energy is the Holy Grail of the universe and of health.

Nikolai A. Kozyrev, energy astrophysicist, proved that scalar energy was responsible for the power generation of the stars in the universe. It has been proven that scalar energy is a phase-conjugated, double-helix spiral waveform and acts upon the ether (fundamental particle of the universe) in order to create physical matter such as the stars. Kozyrev observed that scalar light from the stars far exceeded the accepted speed of light of the electromagnetic energy spectrum. Kozyrev observed that scalar energy emitted from the stars had velocities billions of times greater than the electromagnetic speed of light. Scalar energy pre-exists as a connection between the stars and the earth and that this pre-existing connection is responsible for instantaneous velocity as well as instantaneous communication between the stars and the Earth. The pre-existing connection of the stars with the Earth proves that the universe is a hologram whereby all points are interconnected and therefore instantaneous velocity as well as instantaneous communication in the universe are the norm by way of the scalar energy spectrum. In conclusion, Kozyrev's observations point to the fact that scalar energy transcends time and space as the universe utilizes the Life Force in order to communicate with itself instantaneously. In essence, Kozyrev proved the existence of Quantum Entanglement! Kozyrev also documented that scalar energy had a direct effect upon the weight of an object leading him to conclude that scalar energy is the cause of gravity.

Chapter Nine -The Secret of Life, Longevity, and Anti-Aging

Based on Antoine Priore's Research of the 1960s and 1970s the following attributes of Scalar Energy have been formulated:

1. Scalar energy is a phase-conjugated, double-helix that can reprogram mutated DNA of cancer cells into normal cells. Priore had an almost 100 percent cure rate for all types of cancer in animals and humans.

2. Scalar energy can disassemble viruses, bacteria, fungi, heavy metals, chemicals, vaccines plus any foreign material, which the body can easily dispose of via its macrophage system.

3. Scalar energy can piggy back frequencies imprinting them into fluids.

4. By its ability to imprint frequencies into fluid, scalar energy provides the mechanism for storing memory in the body. Since the body fluid makes up 70 percent of our body, it acts as the antenna for attracting ambient scalar energy from our surroundings to help restore health. Eating raw foods, which stores scalar energy produced by the sun in the form of biophotons, is another source for restoring health.

5. Scalar energy has the ability to make new cells and repair old ones or whatever tissue(s) in the body by stimulating stem cells. In reality, it can transmutate anything that it needs. Thomas Galen Hieronymus in the 1940s proved that transmutation is possible.

6. Each organ or tissue in the body possesses a unique scalar energy harmonic.

7. Broadcasting a reverse-phase angle scalar energy harmonic of a disease back into the body will negate the condition.

In a "Cliff Notes" version, scalar energy enables practitioners to effectively heal pretty much any medical condition by correcting the mutated DNA.

Chapter Nine -The Secret of Life, Longevity, and Anti-Aging

The Energy Cycle of Life

The research done by such geniuses as Antoine Priore, Thomas Galen Hieronymus, Nikola Tesla, Royal Raymond Rife, Georges Lakhosky, Nikolai A. Kozyrev, and Thomas Henry Moray provide the blue print for "The Cycle of Life." Since the closer one gets to the truth, the more simplistic the solution becomes. The following overview is my "Cliff Notes" version.

According to Nikolai Kozyrev, the sun produces scalar energy. The research of Thomas Hieronymus proved that scalar energy is the key component for stimulating photosynthesis. He proved his theory by growing plants in total darkness just by exposing them to scalar energy. Fritz Albert Popp, a German researcher documented that plants store energy in the form of biohotons. Supplements made from a food source have biophotons where as synthetic vitamins do not. Kozyrev showed that scalar energy is a spiraling energy that was the primal force of the universe as well as of all creation. Its waveform is a doulble-helical configuration the same as DNA. In essence, scalar energy provides the template for correcting DNA mutations. Also of importance is the fact that scalar energy has the ability to disassemble viruses, bacteria, heavy metals, chemicals and in reality functions as the ganitorial service of the body. In response to the breakdown of these toxins, the body carries the debris away via the macrophages, polymorphonucleocytes, and other defensive cell types.

Scalar energy can piggyback Rife frequencies and imprint them into water or bodily fluids. This is how our memory system works. Your memory is held in the tissues and fluid of the body. This is borne out when heart transplant patients receive someone else's heart but they also take on the characteristics of the donor, which reveals itself in newly acquired cravings like beer or other foods which they previously never liked.

Chapter Nine -The Secret of Life, Longevity, and Anti-Aging

Connecting the dots makes it possible to now see The cycle of Life. The sun produces the scalar energy. The plants store the scalar energy in the form of biophotons, which are then eaten by humans and animals. The scalar energy is used to repair the body and also provide its memory system. In addition, since the body is made of ninety percent fluid this fluid then becomes the antenna of the body to pull in ambient scalar energy from the environment. Unfortunately, EMFs (wi-fi, cell phone frequencies, TATRA emergency broadband frequencies, etc.), pesticides, heavy metals, viruses and other pathogens act to disrupt our antenna thus diminishing our ability to absorb scalar energy and reduce our body's healing capacity. Our magnificent functioning body is then connected to the universe and all other living beings by means of quantum entanglement. Quantum entanglement's basis is scalar energy, which travels multiple times faster than the speed of light. This is the definition of instantaneous. Because the same thought can be present in two people at the same time. In a nut shell we are all connected. Our thoughts are in the form of scalar energy. This is why we can send healing affirmations to anyone in the world no matter where they are located. It is also the reason why one must be careful for what they wish for. What you put out to the universe positive or negative will come back to you.

Seven Reasons Why Today's Conventional Medicine Is Obsolete

Proponents of conventional medicine continue to espouse their mantra that today's medical concepts represent the "gold standard" in the health industry. The German Minister of Propaganda, Joseph Goebbels was reported to have told Hitler, that if you tell a big enough lie long enough people will believe it and if you continue to tell the same lie you will believe it. When one takes a closer look at what medicine is doing today, one quickly realizes that the American people have been sold an illusion of a "gold standard" which in reality is not only obsolete but dangerous.

Understanding the points presented below supports the premise that it makes no difference which governmental health care coverage is offered because the underlying medical principles of the health care delivery system are based on faulty science, disinformation, invasive procedures, and toxic drug remedies. As Albert Einstein said, "Insanity is doing the same thing over and over again and expecting a different result."

Number 1: Blood Tests

Blood tests used for diagnoses are based on ranges derived from a sick population. True health should be measured against a healthy population. A more logical approach and truer assessment would be to establish ranges based on 1000 healthy people who live a healthy lifestyle (eat organic food, drink clean water, exercise regularly, etc.) Unfortunately, the values would place the majority of our population in the sick range.

A perfect example of the inaccuracy and absurdity of placing diagnostic value in blood testing is a patient, who in 2011, presented himself for a second opinion. His "conventional" medical doctors wanted him to have a liver transplant. His alkaline phosphatase (an enzyme measured in the blood signifying liver or bone damage) was elevated for many years and his liver had been swollen for the past 27 years. Not wanting to take anti-organ rejection medication for the rest of his life was the motivating factor for seeking a second opinion. Quantum Testing Technique diagnosed the presence of benzene and hepatitis B virus in his liver. Seven months later after adhering to a nutritional regime to remove the two offending stressors in his liver, his 27 year swollen liver went back to normal and his alkaline phosphatase also normalized. Blood tests do not reveal the underlying reason for the illness. In reality, it only reveals the body's reaction to the underlying cause(s).

Number 2: Cancer Treatment

The mechanism for cancer was discovered by Otto Warburg, M.D., P.h.D. Doctor Warburg won a Nobel Prize in physiology in 1931 for his incredible discovery. The true cause of cancer is a lack of oxygen. When the cell membranes become altered by the ingestion of adulterated omega-6 oils (corn, safflower, grapeseed, canola, sunflower, and soy), the corrupted cell membrane lacking the omega-6 oils dramatically reduces the influx of oxygen into the cell. Dr. Otto Warburg's discovery showed that when the oxygen level diminished by 35% fermentation occurs in which the glucose converts to lactic acid. Acidifying the internal environment of the cell with reduced oxygen levels triggers off the cancer. In reality, cancer represents the ultimate breakdown of the immune system. Additional factors also contribute to the corruption of the cell membranes and years of exposure to toxins provide the straws that break the camel's back. Examples of toxins include: heavy metals, chemicals, poisons (methyl mercaptan, hydrogen sulfide, and thioethers) released from root canal teeth, vaccines and their toxic fillers, genetically modified foods, radiation from Chernobyl and Fukushima, constant exposure to EMFs (electromagnetic frequencies: cell phone and wi-fi), processed foods, and psychological distress. These initiators coalesce to establish a polluted acidic body terrain, increase cell membrane inflammation and permeability, and depress the immune system. All of the above allow opportunistic organisms to flourish and cause cell mutations.

A study published in August 2003 revealed that of adult cancer in the United States and Australia, the use of chemotherapy, when looking at adjuvant and curative use, provided a cure rate of only 2.1% of the time in the U.S.A. and 2.3% of the time in Australia. In essence, chemotherapy is ineffective 97% of the time and is touted as the "gold standard" of cancer treatment.

Another example of medicine's Neanderthal approach to cancer was a recent patient that was referred to my office because of failed conventional cancer treatment. The patient had cancer in the tip of her right lung. Following the "gold standard" of cancer treatment, doctors cut out the cancerous portion of her right lung. In six months, the cancer came back in the upper portion of her left lung. Not wanting to endure the horrors of surgery again, the patient opted for an integrative approach. Energy medicine was used to diagnose the primary stressors present in the patient's biopsy slides. Testing revealed a pesticide, cytomegalovirus, and mercury in the cancerous lung tissue as presented in the histologic slide. The concept of testing the histologic slide for the initiators of the patient's cancer was recently developed by this author and has been successful in resolving several other cancer cases. Because the patient could not afford an extensive vitamin program, she was placed on just the essential supplements to resolve the three primary stressors. Within six months, the cancer in the upper portion of her left lung disappeared. The body's cells want to go back to normal. If the offending stressors are removed, the body can reset itself to "factory default." The closer one gets to the truth the more simplistic the solution. Unfortunately, when it comes to cancer treatment in America, my clinical experience of over 50 years has shown me that most people diagnosed with the Big C function in fear mode and would rather be killed by a notorious doctor using unsuccessful therapies than be healed by a "quack" using natural remedies.

Number 3: Drug Therapy

The body is not deficient in drugs. Faulty logic focuses on changing the body's chemistry to restore blood values back to "normal." The captains of medical industry have artificially lowered the level of cholesterol so that more statin prescriptions could be written. The Weston Price Foundation established a normal cholesterol range of 200 to 250. The pharmaceutical companies have established normal to be 200 or below. What a great marketing strategy.

Prescription drug spending in the U.S. shot up to about $374 billion in 2014. Statins undoubtedly made up a significant portion ($29 billion) of this spending, and now consumers who take such drugs have much more to worry about than the dent it's making in their wallets.

"High" cholesterol is not a disease but just a reaction. A low functioning thyroid will cause elevated cholesterol. No amount of lowering the cholesterol level will fix an existing hypothyroid problem. This approach is pure insanity. The liver produces 80% of the body's cholesterol. Cholesterol is essential for cleansing the liver cells of toxins. Also cholesterol is the primary organic molecule in your brain, and a major constituent in the mylin sheath around your nerves. In addition, the adrenal cortex produces over sixty different hormones and every one of these sixty plus hormones require a cholesterol base for its production. If the body is in distress, it needs additional adrenal hormones to meet the needs of the body and your cholesterol levels have to rise to meet the demand.

Chapter Ten

Please read the documented side effects of the statin drugs:

Causes dementia: Statins make cells unable to repair properly, create nerve problems, and destroy memory, cause forgetfulness and confusion

Reduce your sex drive

Increase your risk for developing type 2 diabetes and cancer

Statins deplete Coenzyme Q10, which can lead to congestive heart failure

Causes breakdown of muscle tissue (rhabdomyolysis) and pain through out the body

Causes cataracts

Causes fatigue

Cause liver and kidney problems

May speed up the aging process: statin drugs act as cellular poisons that accelerate aging and deactivating DNA repair

Other adverse effects include: nausea, diarrhea, abdominal pain, headaches, rashes, myopathy, muscle aches or weakness, tendon problems, depression, chronic fatigue, heart disease, hypertension, stroke, peripheral neuropathies and can even cause death.

The criminality of the health industry was reinforced by a conversation I had with a medical doctor who worked for a VA hospital. He told me that he had to write a certain number of prescriptions for statin drugs each day. I asked him how he was able to sleep at nights. He never answered me.

Number 4: Contaminated Vaccines

Unknown to our citzens, who believe that the FDA, CDC, and physicians are protecting their health, was a major contamination issue that was suppressed by the CDC and FDA. On July 22, 2009, a special meeting was held with twenty-four leading scientists at the National Institutes of Health to discuss early findings that a newly discovered retrovirus was linked to chronic fatigue syndrome (CFS), prostate cancer, lymphoma, and eventually neurodevelopmental disorders in children. All the vaccines that were being produced on chicken embryos were contaminated with chicken retroviruses. The CDC and FDA knew about this discovery in 1990 and said nothing to alert the public. Why? The reason is simple.

First, the CDC would have lost millions of dollars if they would have had to dispose of the contaminated vaccines. Second, the public would have lost faith in the concept that vaccines were safe and would have resisted future inoculations. Dr. Judy Mikovit's reward for making this incredible discovery was that she was put in jail and bankrupted by the powers that be. For those individuals interested in learning the details, I recommend you read Dr. Mikovit's book, *Plague*. It is despicable that our own governmental agency, the FDA, and an independent corporation, the Center for Disease Control (CDC), both lack academic and moral integrity. For those who are unaware, the CDC is an independent corporation who owns 57 patents on vaccines. This is the major reason why the required vaccine schedule for children keeps increasing. By the year 2025, it has been estimated that the vaccine industry will generate revenues of 100 billion dollars.

Number 5: Faulty Concept of Autoimmune Disease

Did you ever ask yourself why the body in its infinite wisdom would attack itself? The reason is hidden in plain view. The organ being attacked is contaminated. Conventional medicine does not have the understanding nor the diagnostic tools to uncover the stressor(s). No blood test can uncover what's hidden within the tissues or organs. In fact, they do not even know what to look for. It's easier to cover their ignorance by telling an unsuspecting public they have an autoimmune disease.

My own daughter was diagnosed with an "autoimmune" disease, Hashimoto's disease, and her endocrinologist wanted to prescribe Tapazole to suppress her over-active thyroid. I told my daughter not to take the drug and tell her endocrinologist I would treat her autoimmune problem with alternative therapies. The doctor politely told my daughter that alternative treatments do not work. Using Quantum Testing technology, I diagnosed Epstein-Barr virus (EBV) in her thyroid. When tested energetically, both Noni (natural antiviral remedy) and ionic silver tested strong against the EBV. I also loaned her my Rife machine to treat the virus. In three months, my daughter's thyroid was normal, which was verified by the endocrinologist's own blood tests and disappearance of all clinical symptoms. Her endocrinologist was not interested in how I successfully diagnosed and treated her autoimmune disease. Most physicians do not want to be confused with the facts.

Number 6: Misconceptions of Congestive Heart Failure

Conventional medicine views congestive heart failure as an ongoing disease that gets worse over time. This is a false narrative. In reality, congestive heart failure is caused by nutritional deficiencies as well as mercury and other toxins from dental and environmental sources. The heart is the biggest endocrine organ in the body. At the myoneural junctions (where the sympathetic nerves innervate the heart muscle), norepinephrine is produced, which causes the heart to forcibly contract and pump the blood around the entire body. The precursor to norepinephrine is the amino acid tyrosine. It's a no brainer once one knows the pathways.

In the 1980s, my father was in acute congestive heart failure. I gave him 1500 mg of tyrosine along with magnesium, calcium, and potassium orotate and in conjunction with coenzyme Q10, L-carnitine, natural B-complex vitamins plus a protomorphagen (desiccated bovine heart tissue that provides the genetic blue print to repair the heart), Cardio Plus. In one week, his congestive heart failure completely resolved. My father was in an experimental program for cardiac arrhythmias with other CHF patients and placed on experimental drugs. I called the pharmaceutical company about the life expectancy on these experimental medications. They told me on average patient's live approximately two years. All the participants in the study died in two years except my father. Four years later I asked my father's cardiologist if he wanted to know what vitamins I had my father on. He had no interest in the fact that I was able to reverse his congestive heart failure and reduce his medications by seventy-five percent with food based nutrients. It's clear to me why medicine still operates in the dark ages. When you present physicians with clinically proven results, they reject it. The medical schools are no different.

Number 7: Dissemination of False Information

The history of the medical establishment is replete with instances where disinformation has been purposely put out to confuse the public. A primary example is the statement that homeopathy is a pseudoscience and its remedies have been found to be no more effective than placebo. It is interesting to note that The Royal Family of England has supported homeopathy for generations and there is still a court homeopath, Dr. Peter Fisher. He is also Clinical Director and Director of Research at the Royal London Hospital for Integrated Medicine. Doctor Fisher has stated that homeopathy was 'safe,' 'popular with patients' and reduced the need for antibiotics.

Writing in the British Medical Journal, Dr. Fisher further stated that alternative therapies were often 'misunderstood' and questioned research which suggested they only work through a placebo effect. He also pointed to several studies that showed integrating homeopathy with conventional medicines led to better patient outcomes and the reduced use of potentially hazardous drugs.

Governments of today are using homeopathy to prevent, treat, or break epidemics within their countries. Some examples are:

The Indian government controls epidemics of malaria, Japanese encephalitis, dengue fever, and epidemic fever with homeopathy
The Cuban government now depends on homeopathy to manage its leptospirosis epidemics and dengue fever outbreaks
The Brazilian government funded two large trials that successfully reduced the incidence of meningococcal disease in those given the homeopathy prophylactic
The governments of Thailand, Columbia and Brazil use homeopathy to manage dengue fever outbreaks and epidemics

(References and sources for these and other instances are found at: Homeoprophylaxis-Human-Records-Studies-Trials [PDF])

At best, medical students receive three hours of nutritional education in their four years of training. They are taught, incorrectly, that synthetic vitamins are no different from food based supplements. With little to no real background in understanding the principles of natural remedies, medical students are easy prey for this disinformation. The false narrative is then continuously reinforced by the pharmaceutical industry once they become medical practitioners.

Doctor Royal Lee, founder of a food based vitamin company, Standard Process Laboratory, stated "In fact, the Food & Drug laws seem to be suspended where synthetic imitations of good foods are concerned, and actually perverted to prosecute makers and sellers of real products. The synthetic product is always a simple chemical substance, while the natural is a complex mixture of related and similar materials. Pure natural Vitamin E was found three times as potent as pure synthetic Vitamin E. Of course the poisonous nature of the synthetic Vitamin D is well established. WHY DO NOT THE PEOPLE AND MEDICAL MEN KNOW THESE FACTS? Is it because the commercial promoters of cheap imitation food and drug products spend enough money to stop the leaking out of information?" [Lee R. How and Why Synthetic Poisons Sold as Imitations of Natural Foods and Drugs? 1948].

The above seven topics represent only the tip of the iceberg. My brief overview of these issues was designed to whet your appetite to dig deeper into the medical cesspool. Because of the Internet, people around the world are slowly waking up to the benefits of natural healing as opposed to "conventional" medicine's distorted view of how the body works. As the population becomes more aware of medicine's obsolete therapies and failures, the establishment has had to mandate therapies like vaccines in order to get compliance.

My prediction is that the time is quickly approaching when "conventional" medicine will implode because of its out of control corruption, arrogance, pervasive ignorance, and resistance to change.

Former New England Journal of Medicine editor on the corruption of American medicine

Harvard Medical School's Dr. Marcia Angell is the author of *The Truth About the Drug Companies: How They Deceive Us and What to Do About It*. She's also the former Editor-in-Chief at the New England Journal of Medicine, arguably one of the most respected medical journals on earth.

"It is simply no longer possible to believe much of the clinical research that is published, or to rely on the judgment of trusted physicians or authoritative medical guidelines. I take no pleasure in this conclusion, which I reached slowly and reluctantly over my two decades as an editor of The New England Journal of Medicine."

Dr. Marcia Angell

Appendix - A: Theraphi Plasma System

Theraphi Plasma System

Gerald H. Smith, DDS, DNM

303 Corporate Drive East
Langhorne, PA 19047
(800) 272-2323
www.icnr.com

In my 50 years of clinical practice, I have come to the conclusion that the common denominator for achieving real healing and health is with the use of scalar energy. The Theraphi Plasma System, which is now available in our practice, utilizes 18 specific healing frequencies coupled with a Bio-Active Plasma field of energy to effect cellular regeneration. When scalar energy and frequencies are combined their effect is much greater than either one alone. A treatment session takes between 6 and 9 minutes and is totally non-invasive. Repeat sessions can be safely accomplished with only a one-hour hiatus.

An example of Theraphi's incredible effectiveness was recently witnessed when one of my patients who had experienced left knee pain since March 2016 had total resolution in two days with just two five-minute sessions. He had had acupuncture, chiropractic, and massage therapy during the five-month period with no lasting results. Of interest, a decrease in the inflammatory process was documented by means of infrared photography. A dramatic decrease of 11.54^0 F drop in temperature occurred immediately following treatment on the second day. The patient was in awe of the results.

The Theraphi Plasma System integrates the research of Raymond Royal Rife's healing frequencies from the 1930's, Nikola Tesla's non-invasive scalar wave electrotherapy from the 1920's, Antoine Priore's electromagnetic healing technology from the 1960's and '70's, and Georges Lakhovsky, a Russian physicist living in France who integrated the research of the three aforementioned pioneers. The ultimate benefit of the plasma generator is that the coherent electromagnetic field created by the Theraphi System restores your body to its original condition. In other words, your cells revert back to a factory default setting when everything was in a state of health. This represents anti-aging at its finest.

The work of Vlail Kaznacheyev, a Russian researcher in the mid-1970's, showed that the use of scalar electromagnetic waves can reverse cell death and the disease process. Rife, Priore, Lakhovsky, and Kaznacheyev successfully reversed cancers in both animals and humans. By reversing the aging process, this technology has been shown to be effective for:

• Pain reduction
• Reduction of inflammation
• Tissue regeneration
• Enhancing cancer remission
• Anti-aging
• Cell memory reversal

It becomes an obvious conclusion that if a cell that is in a pathologic, abnormal or diseased state can be reversed, then diseases such as MERSA, Alzheimer's, dementia, heart disease, sports and other types of injuries and other medical illnesses can also be reversed.

Why Is Scalar Energy So Effective?

The closer one gets to the truth, the more simplistic the solution. Scalar energy is the Holy Grail of the universe and of health.

Nikolai A. Kozyrev, energy astrophysicist, proved that scalar energy was responsible for the power generation of the stars in the universe. It has been proven that scalar energy is a phase-conjugated, double-helix spiral waveform and acts upon the ether (fundamental particle of the universe) in order to create physical matter such as the stars. Kozyrev observed that scalar light from the stars far exceeded the accepted speed of light of the electromagnetic energy spectrum. Kozyrev also stated that **scalar energy** emitted from the stars had velocities billions of times greater than the electromagnetic speed of light. Scalar energy pre-exists as a connection between the stars and the earth, and this pre-existing connection is responsible for instantaneous velocity as well as instantaneous communication between the stars and the Earth. The pre-existing connection of the stars with the Earth proves that the universe is a hologram whereby all points are interconnected and therefore instantaneous velocity and instantaneous communication in the universe are the norm by way of the scalar energy spectrum. In conclusion, Kozyrev's observations point to the fact that scalar energy transcends time and space as the universe utilizes the Life Force in order to communicate with itself instantaneously. In essence, Kozyrev proved the existence of **Quantum Entanglement**! Kozyrev also documented that scalar energy had a direct effect upon the weight of an object, leading him to conclude that it is the cause of gravity.

Based on Antoine Priore's Research of the 1960's and 70's, the following attributes of Scalar Energy have been formulated:

1. Scalar energy is a phase-conjugated, double-helix that can reprogram mutated DNA of cancer cells into normal cells. Priore had an almost 100 percent cure rate for all types of cancer in animals and humans.
2. Scalar energy can disassemble viruses, bacteria, fungi, heavy metals, chemicals, vaccines plus any foreign material, which the body can easily dispose of via its macrophage system.
3. Scalar energy can piggyback frequencies imprinting them into fluids.
4. By its ability to imprint frequencies into fluid, scalar energy provides the mechanism for storing memory in the body. Since the body fluid makes up 70 percent of our body, it acts as the antenna for attracting ambient scalar energy from our surroundings to help restore health. Eating raw foods, which stores scalar energy produced by the sun in the form of biophotons, is another source for restoring health.
5. Scalar energy has the ability to make new cells and repair old ones or whatever damaged tissue(s) in the body by stimulating stem cells. In reality, it can transmutate anything that it needs. Thomas Galen Hieronymus in the 1940s proved that transmutation is possible.
6. Each organ or tissue in the body possesses a unique scalar energy harmonic.
7. Broadcasting a reverse-phase angle scalar energy harmonic of a disease back into the body will negate the condition.

In a "Cliff Notes" version, scalar energy enables practitioners to effectively heal pretty much any medical condition by correcting the mutated DNA.

Appendix - A1: Theraphi Set-Up

Theraphi Plasma System

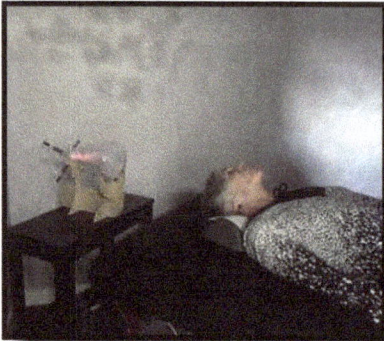

The electronics beneath the table provide a modified Tesla coil to generate a high voltage. Scalar waves plus electromagnetic frequencies are transmitted by the pink glowing inert gases within the plasma tubes. The plasma field surrounds the patient affecting every cell of their body. A healing session lasts for 5 minutes.

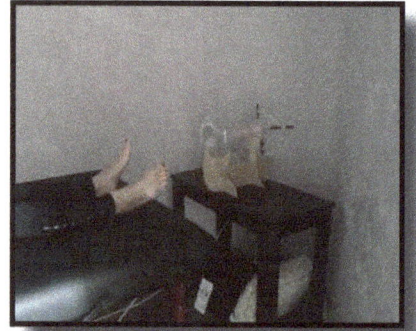

Glass tube filled with inert gases provides the carrier wave to transmit the 18 healing frequencies to the body.

A second glass tube located at the patient's feet enables a fractual wave form (shaped like two acorns) to form around the patient's body.

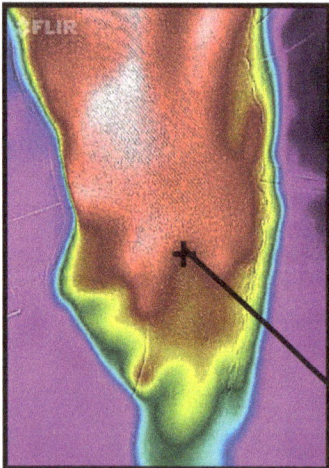

An 11.54°F degree drop in temperature occurred immediately following the second Theraphi Plasma treatment. The patient's five months of constant pain immediately and totally resolved.

Temperature readings were taken at the exact location pre and post treatment.

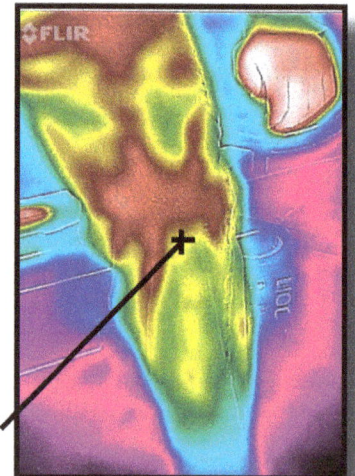

Pre-Tx temperature at the knee was 81.87°F

Post-Tx temperature at the knee was 70.33°F

Appendix - B: CyberScan, Scalar Energy

The CyberScan Professional System is a quantum physics based CE-Class IIa medical device in the EU and FDA registered as neurological biofeedback device. Made 100% in Germany. CyberScan utilizes state-of-the-art proprietary, scalar-energy technology based upon the patents and investigational trials of experimental physicist Nikola Tesla (1856-1943) and P.E.A.R. (Princeton Engineering Anomaly Research).

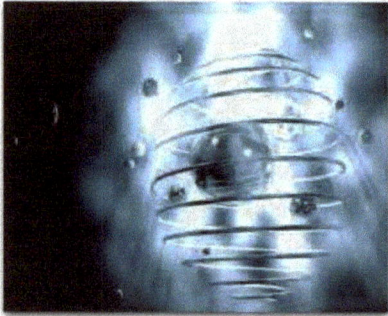

The CyberScan determines your present and past health condition based on the trends that are identified in the current state of the body's immune system. With this data base of information it can predict and modify an individual's personal future health.

Benefits of Cyberscan:

- Reduce stress and anxiety
- Improve athletic performance
- Improve sleep and dream recall
- Enhanced mental clarity
- Reduce depression
- Reduce addictions
- Improved general health
- Reduce aging factors
- Enhanced muscle mobility
- Reduce digestive disorders
- Enhance detoxification

Scalar Energy
The Best Kept Secret
Theraphi System

ADVANTANGES OF SCALAR ENERGY:

- REPAIRS DNA
- DETOX PATHOGENS, CHEMICALS, VACCINES
- ELIMINATE ACUTE AND CHRONIC PAIN
- RESTORES VITALITY OF LIFE
- RESTORES CELLS BACK TO A STATE OF HEALTH
- ELIMINATES HEAVY METALS
- ENHANCES THE HEALING PROCESS

THE BEST OF BOTH WORLDS

The CyberScan System defines the underlying core issues quickly, accurately, non-invasively and helps remove the offending issues.

Scalar Energy restores all the cells, tissues and fluids back to their factory default settings. Combining the two modalities achieves total healing.

GERALD H. SMITH, DDS, DNM
303 CORPORATE DRIVE EAST
LANGHORNE, PA 19047
(215) 968-4324
(800) 272-2323

*Cyberscan and Theraphi are not a diagnostic tool. They are not intended to Diagnose, Treat, or Cure Disease or Illness, nor are they to be presented or construed, in any way, as a substitute for Professional Medical, Surgical or Psychiatric Care or Treatment.

CyberScan Professional System

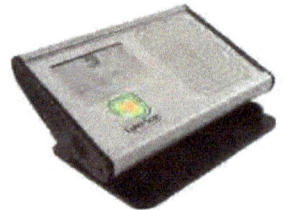

Intelligent Evolution Through Use of Proprietary Scalar Wave Technology

Non-Invasive
Restore Your Vitality
Scientifically Proven Safe

You owe it to yourself and your family to investigate this incredible discovery

Appendix - B: CyberScan, Scalar Energy

10-Second Scan:

CyberScan quickly scans the morphogenetic or energy fields around cells, determines where the stressors are within the body, and creates a 100% natural scalar information carrier that communicates, as well as stimulates, the self-healing properties of the immune system.

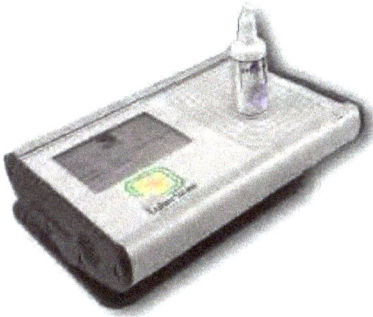

eeCARD:

CyberScan creates a personalized, electro-magnetic protection card designed specifically to protect your immune system from electrosmog and geopathic stress.

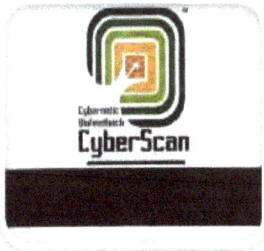

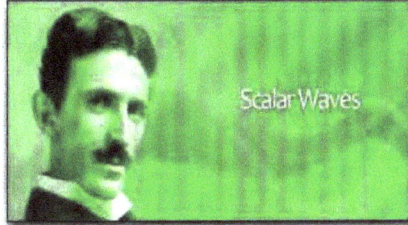

CyberScan Philosophy

During the past 25 years patients have witnessed incredible advances in medical technology which have improved their quality of life. As a result of this intelligent evolution, the CyberScan Professional System evolved. This system has incorporated the genius of Nicola Tesla's discovery of scalar waves and the most advanced concepts of Quantum Physics. The benefits of this integration is that health problems can now be solved more cost effectively. By using non-invasive scalar wave technology practitioners can now correct abnormal energy fields surrounding cells. When the morphogenic or energy field around the cell becomes normalized it communicates this information to the internal parts and reprograms the cell to work normally. When cells function normally the symptoms disappear.

Cyberscan supports and balances the immune system to reduce stress that may be caused by:

- Infections
- Fungi
- Toxic Chemicals
- Pesticides-Herbicides-Insecticides
- Mercury and other Heavy Metals
- Electrosmog
- Geopathic Stress
- Radioactive Elements
- Psyche: Emotional or Mental
- Energetic Distortions
- Teeth

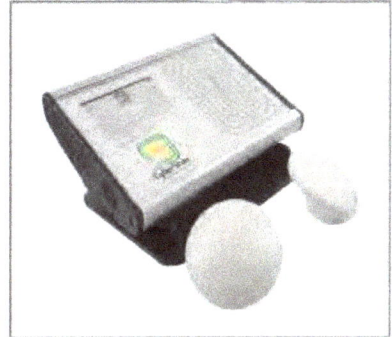

CyberScan's Innovative Healing Process

The CyberScan System approaches health issues in several ways. First phase detects the underlying cause(s) of your problem. This process takes approximately three months. Most patients are seen every two weeks to be rescanned. If your health issues are more serious, you may require more attention on a weekly basis. CyberScan also addresses EMFs (Electromagnetic Frequencies), Wi-Fi, cell phone frequencies and much more. A custom eeCard is specifically programed to meet your needs. By placing this card under the foot of your bed it protects against potentially dangerous frequencies. This "insurance" policy helps you obtain a more restful night sleep. In addition to the card, you will receive a liquid that is programed with healing energy, a direct infusion of frequencies from a specially designed instrument, and an innovative transfer of scalar wave technology during the one to two week interval between visits.

Phase two focuses on regeneration during the second three month period. Once the offending factors are removed the scalar waves start the restoration of normal healthy function.

Invest in your health. Make an appointment now.

Appendix - C: Truth About Taking a Daily Aspirin

Truth About Taking A Daily Aspirin

Tens of millions of Americans take an aspirin a day, mainly for one of two reasons: The most common indication for the widespread use of aspirin is to prevent the clotting of the blood, to help prevent heart attacks and strokes. Second, aspirin is anti-inflammatory and used in the primary prevention of diseases that are thought to be caused by chronic inflammation, including colon cancer.

Six Studies Reveal the INEFFECTIVENESS of Aspirin!

The first study, published in 2010, comes from the journal *Expert Opinion on Pharmacotherapy*. The researchers studied the role of aspirin in the primary prevention of cardiovascular disease in patients with diabetes. These patients were diabetic but had no history or evidence of heart disease. The fact that they had diabetes put them at high risk for heart disease, and aspirin was studied as a low-risk, low-cost primary prevention therapy. The study concluded that "aspirin was ineffective in preventing cardiovascular disease in patients who had diabetes but no existing heart disease at the time.

The second study, also from 2010, comes from the prestigious Journal of the *American College of Cardiology*. The study was designed to determine the outcome for patients who were taking aspirin prior to having a coronary event. The researchers noted the existing "controversy" regarding whether prior aspirin use predicts worse outcomes in patients who go on to experience acute coronary events. The study concluded: Taking aspirin had worse outcomes and a higher risk of having a heart attack than those not taking aspirin—exactly the opposite of what the doctors told them.

The third study, appearing in 2005 in the gold-standard *New England Journal of Medicine*, examined whether aspirin use lowered the risk of cardiovascular disease for women in general. The study concluded: the researchers found a lowered risk for one type of stroke (ischemic, or blood clot, strokes), but aspirin did not affect the overall death rate from cardiovascular events. This study found no clear evidence that aspirin helped prevent hemorrhagic (bleeding) strokes, while another study in the journal Stroke identified clear evidence that, in women, taking aspirin daily increased the risk of both types of strokes. The conclusion stated: at least in women older than age sixty-five, daily aspirin use was shown to increase the risk for strokes.

Studies show that aspirin is far from a benign drug. For example, a 2010 study published in *The American Journal of Medicine* showed that "Regular use of aspirin, NSAIDs [nonsteroidal anti-inflammatory drugs], or acetaminophen (Tylenol) increases the risk of hearing loss in men, and the impact is larger on younger individuals."

A 2009 study from the journal *Current Medical Research and Opinion* found that even low-dose aspirin therapy is associated with significant gastrointestinal toxicity: "Data suggest that acetylsalicylic acid or aspirin causes significant gastroduodenal damage even at the low doses used for cardiovascular protection.

Finally, a 2011 study in Alimentary Pharmacology and Therapeutics linked daily aspirin use with the development of Crohn's disease (CD), an illness becoming increasingly prominent in our medical landscape. The authors reported "a strong positive association between regular aspirin use and CD" (but not ulcerative colitis).

SAFER ALTERNATIVES
Are there alternatives to low-dose aspirin therapy? Many natural medicines inhibit platelet aggregation, thin the blood and reduce inflammation without any of the risks incurred from low-dose aspirin therapy.

- Nattokinase or lumbrokinase, both enzymes have shown anti-clotting effects as well as heart-strengthening properties.
- A 1999 study showed that pycnogenol, the French pine bark extract, not only inhibited platelet aggregation in smokers (a high-risk group) as effectively as aspirin, but also did it without adversely affecting bleeding time.

- Zymessence: Pharmaceutical grade systemic enzyme that digests all foreign protein in the blood. It is also anti-inflammatory with no side effects.
- Turmeric
- Ginger
- Cayenne pepper
- Garlic
- Cassia cinnamon
- Ginkgo bloba
- Grape seed extract
- Vitamin E (delta tocopherol)
- Bromelain
- Omega-3 and Omega-6 fats

Appendix - D: Liver Detox

Detoxing the liver

Written by Kathryn Alexander and edited by Gerald H. Smith, DDS, DNM

The conclusion that nowadays treatment follows the premise "the more that is wrong with you, the more you put in." Many patients come with a bag full of nutritional supplements, vitamins, homeopathic remedies and herbal preparations and have been following a diet that I couldn't fault on a scientific nutritional basis and yet they have seen no significant impact on health or real reversal of their condition. Why, they ask. The answer is simple: if you don't address the toxicity then you cannot expect long-term results. In fact, with detoxification – the more that is wrong with you, **the less you put in**. *Releasing the toxic load occurs once you take the pressure off the system, not by putting more pressure on the system, particularly using products that force an action.*

When assessing a patient's degree of toxicity there are three questions that need to be answered: how great is the toxic load, how well can it be eliminated to the outside and how fast can we safely do this? Although a person may come with specific problems in reality these only reflect varying degrees of toxicity. The more toxic, the lower the vitality and the more severe the illness. In any case history you see a gradual deterioration on all levels; the impairment of the digestive system, which may have started with simple food intolerances but progressed to severe allergies and chemical sensitivities; the gradual impairment of the immune system giving rise to recurrent infection, candidiasis and later parasites; the gradual decline of thyroid activity (closely connected with immune function) where the slight drop in body temperature allows persistent activation of viruses including HIV; poor blood sugar control leading to addictions and later depression and last, but not least, the general decline in fertility.

So how does one handle toxicity and remove it? Detoxification involves first getting the cells to release toxicity and second, ensuring its elimination to the outside. The *second part of the equation is the most important* of all for you **may be unleashing years of accumulated toxins** that have been "safely" tucked away (albeit lowering the vitality of the tissues) into the circulation at one hit. **This can be a greater toxic insult to the tissues and organs than the small doses received on a daily basis** and **may leave the body in a more weakened condition than before as the toxins will merely redistribute**, perhaps in more vulnerable organs, such as the brain. Unfortunately this can be the first mistake practitioners make. They feel that the greater the toxicity, the more aggressive the treatment should be. *Any treatment that aims to shift toxins from the cells but does not factor in their final elimination via the liver can have disastrous consequences.*

On the other hand, many people may opt to fast in the belief that this will provoke the greatest detoxification. Although fasting does reduce the burden from the system, *in a nutritionally deficient body, where there are no reserves, it can lead to deterioration. Fasting may not provoke a detoxification by itself as the body drops into a go slow mode and shuts down its metabolism - this includes the capacity for detoxification.* A recent case I had provides a fine example of the famous saying by the late Dr. Christopher who said "Fasting is like fire – it can either gently warm you or it can kill you."

A 47 year old man suffering with chronic fatigue over the last four years sold his business and decided to take a six week holiday and go on a water fast. His previous history showed that he suffered tonsillitis as a child, later developed food intolerances, hay fever, and recently had suffered gall stones. There was a very strong family history of heart conditions and cancer. Almost immediately following the fast the man was diagnosed with bacterial endocarditis which carries a 30% mortality. He underwent treatment but was left with a permanently compromised a heart valve where he may require a valve replacement within the next 2 years.

All detoxification programs are alkaline-forming, which means that they are high in vegetables and fruits and low in fats and protein. **The higher the volume of raw vegetables and fruits, juiced, and the greater their ratio to protein and fats, the more aggressive the cleanse. By reducing the ratio and adding cooked vegetables and small amounts of protein, we reduce the rate of detoxification, and in a very toxic body a period of loosening and slow elimination may be more appropriate than an aggressive cleanse, particularly if there is known to be a high volume of toxins in the system.**

When such poisons are unlocked in our system we must ensure their removal to the outside or they will damage the body and leave it not only vulnerable to opportunistic infection but also the progression of any existing disease process. We assume that the body is able to keep pace with our detoxification requirements on a day by day basis, removing toxins as fast as they come in. In truth, **the combination of our toxic exposure with a nutritionally depleted state can erode the vitality and depress our capacity to detoxify adequately. Toxins can be stored for decades, and can be very difficult to remove.** This has been very apparent in my own work with cancer patients. It can take around five months on a strong program (such as the Gerson TherapyTM) for a patient who has had chemotherapy to begin releasing the drug residue. As the elimination begins, we see similar symptoms that resulted from the initial treatment. In particular we see suppression of the bone marrow as the drug residue is shifted into the circulation; t*he patient is effectively getting a second dose.* If this is managed properly then no ill-effects occur.

So the more toxic the patient becomes, the more "stuck" they are and the treatment must be more carefully managed. The liver is like an exit ramp from a congested freeway. If the ramp is blocked, the traffic will jam. If we decide to send in a bulldozer to shift the traffic you will have a pile up. This is exactly what happens when one detoxifies too aggressively without ensuring that the liver can cope with the amount of toxicity released. The liver is like a filter which can clog and become weakened. This is especially true if you have suffered from any chronic infection (glandular fever, Ross River Fever, hepatitis, digestive problems and gall stones).

One needs to support the liver in its task of detoxification and there are various ways to do this. One can take specific herbs and vitamins, which promote the production and flow of bile by the liver (major route of detoxification of drugs and chemicals) but this may not be totally effective as a good proportion of the toxic bile is reabsorbed from the gastrointestinal tract. Use of the coffee enema is a miraculous little method used by Dr. Max Gerson in his famous cancer therapy. Dr. Gerson's genius lay in the fact that he recognized the dangers of a poorly managed toxic release into the system and he found a way to deal with it. As he was working against time with many of his terminally ill patients, it was vital that he secured maximum detoxification right from the beginning. Dr. Gerson found that if he matched the rate of elimination of toxicity from the tissues with it's rate of removal to the outside, then over time total healing occurred. It was the coffee enema that made this possible.

Dr. Gerson knew that the coffee enema dilated the bile ducts and caused a flushing of toxic bile from the liver. (Drinking coffee constricts the bile ducts). He also knew that this was the most effective method for detoxification. Since Dr. Gerson's time, various active ingredients in coffee have been identified and most interestingly, the palmitates present in coffee enhance by 7-fold the ability of the enzyme, glutathione S transferase to bind and eliminate toxic elements in the bile. Furthermore, this activity in the small intestine **does not allow for the reabsorption of the toxic bile**. Most cholerectic substances (stimulate flow of bile: menthol, ginger, Gentian root, Bupleurum root, red beet leaves and beet juice, Swedish bitters [angelica root, carline thistle root, camphor, manna, myrrh, rhubarb root, saffron, senna, theriac venetaian, zedoary root]), although they may increase the bile flow, do not ensure a complete removal of toxins; they work very slowly, and are unable to help the liver accommodate any increased requirements during heavy detoxification.

 To assist detoxification the coffee enema is recommended. It guards against a toxic buildup that can make you feel so sick and in this way help the body to heal. Full details on how to prepare and administer the coffee enema are found in my book Reversing Cancer. It is important to remember that the coffee enemas go hand-in-hand with the juices: no enemas – no juices and no juices – no enemas. The juices help shift toxicity from the tissues and the coffee enema ensure it's removal to the outside. If used without the juices they will ultimately deplete nutrients. The rule of thumb is 3 juices (3 x 250mls) per coffee enema. If you increase the juices then you can safely increase the enemas.

Bile acids are made in the liver by the cytochrome P450-mediated oxidation of cholesterol. They are conjugated with taurine or the amino acid glycine, or with a sulfate or a glucuronide, and are then stored in the gallbladder, which concentrates the salts by removing the water. In humans, the rate limiting step is the addition of a hydroxyl group on position 7 of the steroid nucleus by the enzyme cholesterol 7 alpha-hydroxylase. Upon eating a meal, the contents of the gallbladder are secreted into the intestine, where bile acids serve the purpose of emulsifying dietary fats. Bile acids serve other functions, including eliminating cholesterol from the body, driving the flow of bile to eliminate catabolites from the liver, emulsifying lipids and fat soluble vitamins in the intestine to form micelles that can be transported via the lacteal system, and aiding in the reduction of the bacteria flora found in the small intestine and biliary tract.

Cholic acid is a bile acid, a white crystalline substance insoluble in water (soluble in alcohol and acetic acid), with a melting point of 200-201 °C. Salts of cholic acid are called cholates. Cholic acid, along with chenodeoxycholic acid, is one of two major bile acids produced by the liver where it is synthesized from cholesterol. Of the two major bile acids, cholate derivatives represent approximately eighty percent of all bile acids. These derivatives are made from cholyl-CoA which forms a conjugate with either glycine, or taurine, yielding glycocholic and taurocholic acid respectively.

Cholic acid and chenodeoxycholic acid are the most important human bile acids.

Choline is essential to metabolize fat, cholesterol, proteins, and carbohydrates, effectively. Choline has been shown to be an essential component in promoting liver and gallbladder function and maintaining the integrity of cell membranes. Choline normalizes homocysteine levels in people who have elevated blood homocysteine.

Soybean oil contains a group of compounds called phytosterols, which help maintain the normal balance of LDL (bad) cholesterol to HDL (good) cholesterol in the blood.

Lecithin is converted by the body into choline, a substance that maintains proper liver activity and functions in the transport of fats out of the liver, especially under conditions of stress. Lecithin helps maintain normal cholesterol levels in individuals who have healthy levels.

Dandelion Root contains sesquiterpene lactones, phenolic acids, triterpenes, sterols, vitamins, minerals and other substances that together support healthy liver and gallbladder function by supporting bile production to digest fats, and by assisting the liver in natural filtration and neutralization of accumulated toxins.

Cayenne pepper helps stimulate gastric juice output and cleanses the digestive tract.

Spanish black radish contains unique phytochemicals that stimulate enzymatic activity required to support liver detoxification.

SOD (Superoxide Dismutase) has the highest concentration within the liver than any other organ. An excellent source is pomegranate. An adequate supply insures the liver's ability to detox chemicals, heavy metals and metabolic breakdown of drug products.

The natural B-complex vitamins permits the liver to also breakdown chemicals and metabolic transition compounds. A good natural source is rice.

Turmeric: Turmeric's principal compound, curcumin, is one of the most researched of all the spice compounds. Much of the research and interest in curcumin has centered on its role in preventing and treating breast cancer, but it has also been found to have protective effects against cancers of the bladder, stomach, uterus and cervix. When measured against other phytochemicals, curcumin exhibits at least a ten times greater chemoprotective potency against cancer than its closest rivals.

Turmeric and Cancer

Curcumin is known to protect against cancer through the following mechanisms.

- Assists the body's natural tumor-suppressing mechanisms.
- Destroys cancer cells by stimulating apoptosis (programmed cell death) in these cells thereby terminating the immortality so typical of cancer cell lines.
- Halts tumor proliferation by inhibiting DNA synthesis in the cancer cells and disrupting their replication.
- Inhibits the formation of the abnormal blood vessels that are essential for tumour growth.

One of turmeric's most promising uses is in the prevention and treatment of breast cancer. Most breast cancers are hormone dependent, requiring estrogen as a growth stimulant. Tamoxifen, which is one of the most used drugs in the treatment of breast cancer, works against this hormone-mediated process, interfering with estrogen's tumor stimulating effects. Curcumin exhibits its anti-estrongenic effects by blocking the estrogen-dependent receptors on tumor cells, thereby interrupting the stimulatory effects of estrogen and slowing tumor growth. Curcumin may be at least as effective as tamoxifen as an estrogen antagonist, with none of the attendant side effects of this drug.

Radiotherapy and chemotherapy are widely used, but imperfect treatments for cancer. Not only do they have serious, debilitating side effects, but tumor cells often develop resistance to these therapeutic modalities. They also activate COX-2 enzymes that are part of the inflammatory process underlying many cancers. Turmeric reduces the activation of COX-2 enzymes and sensitizes the tumor cells to both radiotherapy and chemotherapy, enhancing their therapeutic effects.

Apart from curcumin, other phytochemicals found in turmeric are also known to have chemoprotective effects. Therefore, when it comes to prevention, it is better to take the parent spice, turmeric, rather than the pure curcumin extract. However, the treatment of existing breast cancer may call for more specific dosages of curcumin, the administration of which would need to be supervised by a qualified health practitioner.

Alzheimer's (AD) and Parkinson's Diseases

Curcumin exhibits several properties that make it a valuable preventive agent for these two devastating and increasingly common diseases. Although turmeric is probably most effective as a preventive agent against these illnesses, it may also help by improving cognitive problems and inhibiting further deterioration of existing disease.

Curcumin works against neurodegenerative diseases via the following mechanisms:

- The accumulation of amyloid protein in the brain is an important factor associated with Alzheimer's disease. Its deposition is associated with oxidative damage and inflammation in the brain tissues. Curcumin is both a potent antioxidant and anti-inflammatory agent and has been shown to suppress oxidative damage, inflammation and the deposition of damaging amyloid protein in the brain. It is possible that it may actually disaggregate existing amyloid plaques and, in so doing, could possibly reverse the course of the disease.
- Another cause of amyloid deposition in the brain is probably due to the accumulation of certain metals, as higher concentrations of harmful metals have been found in the brains of AD sufferers that in non-AD individuals. Metal molecules that find their way into the brain can both induce amyloid aggregation and are directly toxic to brain cells. Certain chelating agents have shown promise in the treatment of Alzheimer's disease and curcumin's chelating properties enable it to assist the body in the removal of potentially toxic metals from the brain and other tissues.
- The abnormal proliferation of the brain's non-neuronal cells is another pathological process that is associated with the development of both Alzheimer's and Parkinson's diseases. Curcumin prevents the proliferation of these cells which, if allowed to continue growing, cause damage to the brain's neuronal tissue.

Inflammatory Diseases

Much of turmeric's anti-inflammatory potency can be attributed to curcumin, which is both an effective COX-2 inhibitor as well as a strong antioxidant. However, other phytochemicals found in turmeric, in particular the salicylates, also make a valuable contribution to its anti-inflammatory activities and thereby its preventive properties against arthritis, autoimmune disorders and the general health consequences of chronic systemic inflammation and degenerative diseases.

Chelation

Copper and iron are both essential nutrients but if they accumulate in excessive quantities they can cause serious and sometimes irreversible inflammatory and oxidative damage to a variety of tissues. Curcumin is a powerful chelating agent for both metals, binding to the metal ions and allowing them to be safely excreted in the urine.

Traditional use and modern scientific research have shown that turmeric is one of the most valuable spices in our arsenal of disease fighting foods. Synergism between different spices enhances the bioavailability of important compounds such as curcumin. Therefore, to obtain optimum benefit from turmeric, it is important to take it with other common spices.

Those who are serious about maintaining a healthy lifestyle in order to enjoy a good quality of life and reduce the risk of acquiring conditions like Alzheimer's disease and cancer would do well to ensure a daily intake of this golden spice.

Milk Thistle:

What are the health benefits of milk thistle?

Milk thistle has been used for centuries for the treatment of liver disease. Milk thistle appears to be safe and have multiple health benefits on various liver conditions; the available evidence on the mechanisms of action appears promising [1]. Traditionally, milk thistle is commonly used for liver cirrhosis, alcoholic hepatitis, alcoholic fatty liver, liver poisoning, and viral hepatitis.

What ingredients in milk thistle contribute to its beneficial effects?

Milk thistle extracts are standardized to a concentration of 70-80% of flavone lignans including isosilybinin, silybinin, silychristin, and silydianin, which are collectively called silymarin. Silymarin may play a role in displacing toxins binding to the liver and causing the liver cells to regenerate at a faster rate.

Milk thistle is a flowering herb. Silymarin can be extracted from the seeds (fruit). The seeds are used to prepare capsules containing powdered herb or seed; extracts; and infusions (strong teas). [NCCAM]

How do suppliers talk about health benefits of milk thistle?

Milk Thistle has been marketed as an herbal supplement having a protecting benefits on the liver, they claim milk thistle can even regenerate the liver cells in most liver diseases such as cirrhosis, jaundice and hepatitis (inflammation of the liver), cholangitis (inflammation of bile ducts resulting in decreased bile flow). Milk Thistle is also marketed as a preventative medicine to protect each cell of the liver from incoming toxins and encourage the liver to cleanse itself of damaging substances, such as alcohol, drugs, medications, mercury and heavy metals. Milk thistle is also promoted as an agent which can cleanse and detoxify overburdened and stagnant livers, strengthen and tonify weak livers.

Milk thistle is also suggested to be used as a gentle and mild laxative, as it may be able to increase bile secretion and flow in the intestinal tract. This herb is also claimed to be able to lubricate and soften the stools to a mild laxative effect- a balance between constipation and diarrhea. However, scientific supports to these claims are limited. In the following section, we review what scientists found about milk thistle - benefits and side effects.

MILK THISTLE EXTRACT HEALTH BENEFITS; RESEARCH FINDS

Milk thistle silymarin has anti-inflammatory, cytoprotective, and anticarcinogenic effects. These effects are probably related to inhibition of activation of NF-kappa B and the kinases. [7]

ANTI-MICROBIAL ACTIVITIES Milk thistle silybin inhibited RNA and protein synthesis on gram-positive bacteria. [8]

ANTI-OXIDANT Milk thistle, silymarin, reduced NO production at less than 300 ppm. [9]

ARTHEROSCLEROSIS Milk thistle and lecithin have found to have anti-atherosclerotic activity in rabbits. Milk thistle-phospholipid complex showed a strong anti-atherosclerotic activity. [10]

CANCER Milk thistle silymarin exerts chemopreventive effects against tumorigenicity by inhibiting endogenous tumor promoter TNF alpha. [11] Milk thistle silibinin and milk thistle silymarin, have shown the anticancer effects in different cancer cells in multiple studies:

BLADDER Milk thistle silibinin modulates cyclin-dependent kinase inhibitors - cyclin-dependent kinases -cyclin cascade and activates caspase 3 causing growth inhibition and apoptotic death of human bladder transitional cell carcinoma cells. [12] In another study, milk thistle silibinin decreased survivin levels and caspases-PARP cleavages, in accord with a strong apoptotic death and growth inhibition of Human bladder transitional-cell papilloma cells. [13] And, milk thistle silymarin was found to be effective in preventing OH-BBN-induced bladder carcinogenesis in mice. [14]

BREAST An in vitro study has suggested a possible synergism between milk thistle silibinin and conventional cytotoxic agents for breast cancer treatment. [15] Milk thistle extract may exert a strong anticarcinogenic effect against breast cancer involving inhibition the threshold kinase activities of cyclin-dependent kinases and associated cyclins, leading to a G1 arrest in cell cycle progression. [16].

COLON Study showed a chemopreventive ability of milk thistle silymarin against chemically induced colon tumorigenesis.[17]

ENDOTHELIAL CELLS Milk thistle silibinin may exert, at least partly, its anti-cancer effect by inhibiting angiogenesis through induction of endothelial apoptosis via modulation of NF-kappaB, Bcl-2 family and caspases. [18] Milk thistle silibinin toxicity to cancer cells is found to involve the epidermal growth factor receptor signaling pathway. [19]

LUNG Milk thistle containing Silibinin exerted a dose-dependent inhibitory effect on the invasion and motility of human lung cancer cells.[20]

LIVER Milk thistle may be useful in the prevention or treatment of liver dysfunction in patients undergoing anticancer therapy.[21]

PROSTATE In prostate cancer, milk thistle silibinin exerts its anti-cancer effect probably via epidermal growth factor receptor, insulin-like growth factor receptor type I and nuclear factor kappa B signaling [23] Milk thistle extracts possess anticancer activities on human prostate carcinoma. Isosilybin A and B might be the most effective suppressors of prostate-specific antigen secretion by androgen-dependent LNCaP cells. Researchers suggested that milk thistle extracts enriched for isosilybin A or B might possess improved potency in prostate cancer prevention and treatment. [22] Finally, milk thistle silibinin was found to able to down regulate 5alpha-dihydrotestosterone, thus, milk thistle may be beneficial to prostate health.
[23] **There are eight more studies showing milk thistle benefits on prostate [24-32].**

SKIN In studies of rats, milk thistle extracts provided substantial protection against different stages of UVB-induced carcinogenesis, possibly via its strong antioxidant properties. [33] In another study, topical treatment of milk thistle silymarin inhibited 7,12-dimethylbenz(a)anthracene-initiated and several tumor promoters in mouse models. [34] There are two more studies showing the anti-tumor activities of milk thistle extracts on skin cancer: [35]

TONGUE Feeding of milk thistle silymarin (500 p.p.m.) during the promotion phase of 4-NQO-induced rat tumorigenesis exerts chemopreventive ability against tongue squamous cell carcinoma through modification of phase II enzymes activity, cell proliferation, and/or PGE(2) content. [36]

CHOLESTASIS Milk thistle prevents cholestasis induced by estrogens and taurolithocholate via inhibiting cAMP-phosphodiesterase. [38] In 1985, Koch HP reported that milk thistle was a very potent inhibitor of cyclic AMP phosphodiesterase. Milk thistle's constituents, silybin, silydianin and silychristin, are 12.66 to 52.06 times more active than theophylline. [37]

DIABETES Milk thistle extracts may be useful in treatment of non-insulin-dependent diabetes mellitus, as silibinin inhibits glucose-stimulated insulin release in vitro, while not affecting blood glucose concentration in vivo. [39]Aqueous extracts of milk thistle exhibit potent hypoglycaemic and anti-hyperglycaemic activities in normal and streptozotocin diabetic rats without affecting insulin secretion. [40]

HEART Milk thistle extract, silymarin, protects cardiomyocytes against doxorubicin-induced oxidative stress via cell membrane stabilization effect, radical scavenging and iron chelating potency. {41}

IMMUNE MODULATION

A study of mice showed milk thistle silymarin could prevent UVB-induced immuno-suppression and oxidative stress probably by inhibiting the infiltration of leukocytes, and myeloperoxidase activity. [42]

A study demonstrated that milk thistle was immunostimulatory in vitro. Milk thistle increased lymphocyte proliferation in both mitogen and MLC assays. These effects of Milk Thistle were associated with an increase in interferon gamma, interleukin (IL)-4 and IL-10 cytokines in the MLC (table). This immunostimulatory effect increased in response to increasing doses of Milk Thistle. [43]

LIVER

CIRRHOSIS A double blind study of 170 patients with cirrhosis demonstrated that silymarin (milk thistle extract) treatment was effective in patients with alcoholic cirrhosis. [44] A study has suggested that milk thistle and S-adenosylmethionine may be effective in alcoholic cirrhosis. [45]

FIBROSIS Milk thistle silymarin retarded the development of alcohol-induced hepatic fibrosis in 12 baboons, consistent with several positive clinical trials. [46]

INJURY The hepatoprotective properties of milk thistle extracts in acute and chronic liver injury is probably related to inhibition of leukotriene B (4) formation by silibinin [Milk thistle]. [47]

The protective effects of milk thistle on liver injury may be related to the recovery of the membrane fluidities of liver microsome and mitochondria [48]

HEPATITIS C A double-blinded trial of 141 subjects demonstrated that milk thistle extract, silymarin, could improve symptoms and general well-being of patients suffered from hepatitis C. [49] However, some researchers found that milk thistle extracts had no benefits on liver health. For instance, milk thistle extract was found to have no hepatoprotective effect on dairy cows. [50]

NERVOUS SYSTEM

In a cell study, milk thistle silymarin significantly inhibited the LPS-induced activation of microglia and the production of inflammatory mediators, such as tumour necrosis factor-alpha and nitric oxide (NO), and reduced the damage to dopaminergic neurons.[51]

Milk thistle extract protected cultured rat hippocampal neurons against oxidative stress-induced cell death. [52]

MILK THISTLE DRUG INTERACTION

Milk thistle decreased the trough concentrations of indinavir in humans. [53] However, another study showed milk thistle had no apparent effect on indinavir plasma concentrations. [54] This conflicting data might be due to different milk thistle product preparation, extraction method, product composition, experimental design or even the purity of milk thistle.

MILK THISTLE SIDE EFFECTS

Milk thistle appears to be safe and accepted by patients. Only a few cases of milk thistle side effect have been reported. Citations about milk thistle side effects and safety issues from various researchers are summarized as follows:

[1] Silymarin (milk thistle) with few side effects that has been safely used for centuries to treat liver ailments. [55]

[2] Silymarin (milk thistle) side effects include gastrointestinal disturbances and allergic skin rashes.[56]

[3] In a study of 170 patients with cirrhosis, researchers observed no milk thistle side effect. [57]

[4] Silymarin (milk thistle) exposure did not produce any signs of overt toxicity or any changes in relative organ weights. Johnson VJ et al, Physiological responses of a natural antioxidant flavonoid mixture, silymarin, in BALB/c mice: III. [58]

[5] Treatment with milk thistle appears to be safe and well tolerated. No reduction in mortality, but improvements in histology and in biochemical markers of liver function among patients with chronic liver disease were found with milk thistle supplement. [59]

[6] Milk thistle was not associated with a significantly increased risk of adverse events. [60]

[7] High dose of milk thistle may stimulate inflammatory process (from a mice study). [61]

Note: Milk thistle can produce allergic reactions, which tend to be more common among people who are allergic to plants in the same family (e.g. ragweed, chrysanthemium, marigold, and daisy}.

Lipoic Acid: (RLA) is one of the most important and exciting new nutraceutical compounds to hit the market. It is a powerful antioxidant, a critical co-factor in ATP production, regulates lipid and carbohydrate metabolism, signal transduction and gene transcription. Lipoic Acid is also neuroprotective, chelates heavy metals, can reverse enzyme and DNA oxidative damage and crosses the blood brain barrier.

Alpha-lipoic acid, also known as thioctic acid, is a naturally occurring compound that is synthesized by plants and animals, including humans. Alpha-lipoic acid contains two sulfur molecules that can be oxidized or reduced. This feature allows alpha-lipoic acid to function as a cofactor for several important enzymes as well as a potent antioxidant.

DHLA (dihydrolipoic acid) is superior to alpha-lipoic acid (ALA) or R-lipoic acid in free radical quenching capacity – and thus can deliver more comprehensive reduction of oxidative stress for literally EVERY organ and gland, especially the brain and the nervous system. Provides significant help for immune-related concerns, especially fatigue and muscle aches. Now contains resveratrol for unparalleled DNA repair and protection. **

- Nerve and Brain Cell Nourishment, protection and rejuvenation
- Boosts memory, metabolism and ATP synthesis while decreasing oxidative stress
- Significant help for immune related concerns, especially fatigue and muscle aches
- The Ultimate Anti-oxidant capable of quenching every known free radical in living cells, one of the major causes of chronic health dysfunction
- DHLA recycles all major antioxidants, including CoQ-10, glutathione and vitamins E and C

The following are just a few uses for Stabilized DHLA:
Scavenge free radicals, kidney protection, arsenic protection, cadmium protection, mercury protection, restoration of metabolism and mobility, decrease stress on heart, type II diabetes, glaucoma, cataracts , DNA and nerve protection, brain fog, chronic fatigue, nerve function, and much more.

Contains Resveratrol:

- Activates the "longevity gene" known to prolong life and health.
- Inhibits destructive cell activity, also reverses the disease process.
- Protects against cardiovascular disease.
- Reverses arterial damage and age-related illnesses.
- Outperforms Viagra's circulatory effect, boosts Nitric Oxide.
- Buys the cell more time for DNA repair.
- Clears the cell of DNA debris up to 60%.
- A natural anti-inflammatory agent and a powerful antioxidant.

Arsenic Protection: Research has shown that ALA can protect mice from poisoning by sodium arsentie, and arsenical herbicide, insecticide and rodenticide by a ratio of ALA to arsentite of at least 8:1. The mice were protected even if the administration of ALA was given after onset of severe symptoms of poisoning.

Appendix - E: PRESCRIPT-ASSIST™ PROBIOTIC-PREBIOTIC
TREATMENT FOR BACTERIAL-DIARRHEA

PRESCRIPT-ASSIST™ PROBIOTIC-PREBIOTIC TREATMENT FOR BACTERIAL-DIARRHEA: *CLINICAL EXPERIENCE IN ECUADOR*

Alvah C. BITTNER, PhD, CPE[1,2]   **Dra. Rocio CAICEDO, B.**[3]

Dr. Telmo DE la TORRE, C.[4,5]   **Titut N. YOKELSON, PhD**[6]

[1]*Bittner & Associates, Kent, WA, USA*   [2]*Univ. of Washington, Seattle, WA, USA*
[3]*FUNDBASIC, Quito, EC*   [4]*Centro Médico San Pedro, EC*
[5]*Centro De DMPA, San Pedro, EC*   [6]*Nutrit. Labs. Inter., Missoula, MT, USA*

Clinical research was conducted to evaluate the efficacy of *Prescript-Assist*[TM] (P-A), an advanced probiotic-prebiotic formulation for treatment of human bacterial-diarrhea in two communities in Ecuador. P-A has previously demonstrated efficacy against: Canine bacterial-diarrhea in short-term studies; and Irritable-Bowel-Syndrome and related gastric diseases in both short-term and longer-term human studies (e.g., 1-year follow-up). In this study, P-A treatment was shown to result in significantly shorter diarrhea-durations than standard-antibiotics used in treating bacterial diarrhea [$\chi2(4) = 41.1$, $P<2.6\cdot10^{-7}$]. *Prescript-Assist*[TM] and other advanced probiotic-prebiotic combinations have considerable promise as emerging treatments for a wide spectrum of both acute and chronic GI diseases.

INTRODUCTION

This report describes our recent clinical experience using an advanced probiotic-prebiotic formulation for treatment of human bacterial-diarrhea in Ecuador [*Prescript-Assist*[TM] (P-A): Safer Medical, Inc. (SMI), Ft. Benton, MT].[1] The P-A complex previously was found particularly effective for the treatment of a wide variety of human GI disorders and bacterial diarrhea.[1,2,3,4] The particular breadth of efficacy – relative to earlier probiotic treatments – is attributed to the actions of a unique complex of >29 probiotic *soil-based-organisms* (SBOs) and *leonardite*, a prebiotic mix of humic substances that differentially enhance SBO proliferation.[1] Among conditions initially reported as clinically responding to the P-A probiotic-prebiotic complex were both: "Occasional diarrhea" (e.g., travelers); and "Chronic diarrhea" such as associated with Irritable Bowel Syndrome (IBS) and Colitis.[4] Early clinical reports[4] prompted a formal randomized, placebo-controlled, double-blind clinical study with regard to IBS.[3] This placebo-controlled study identified 3 relatively-independent *subsyndromic factors* of IBS: *General ill-feelings/nausea, Indigestion/flatulence*, and *Colitis*. More importantly, the combined probiotic-prebiotic treatment (P-A, 550mg BID) was associated with broad reductions in each of the subsyndromic factors (*Ps* <0.04) – and their associated symptoms – in a two-week double-blind study in patients with IBS.[1]

The reduction in "Colitis" – associated in the literature with a *C. difficile* infection – arguably supported the earlier indications of P-As potential as a treatment for occasional diarrhea.[5] This, together with the earlier clinical observations, encouraged both: Follow-up of P-A's efficacy in the IBS study population[2] and Evaluation of P-A's specific efficacy for bacterial-diarrhea in animal patients.[3] In the remainder of this section, the results of these efforts are introduced both as part of the "background" for the current effort and to set the stage for the "purpose."

---

[1] E-mail address: george@safermedicalinc.com

BACKGROUND

Bacterial diarrhea is one of the most common maladies faced by medical care-givers working in the third-world. In humans, and their canine companions, a number of bacteria have been commonly associated with diarrhea, including: *Salmonella, C. perfringens*, and *C. difficile*. However, these and a variety of other organisms are not uncommonly a part of "healthy intestinal microflora." Hence, stool studies and related diagnostic approaches may be neither timely nor useful when faced with an accelerating outbreak of diarrhea in a closed population. Medical emphases consequently include: immediate treatment to limit the duration of diarrhea; and other actions to limit its possible transmission (particularly as untreated-diarrhea is associated with up to 20% deaths in the young).

The seriousness of bacterial diarrhea and earlier reports of efficacy against "occasional diarrhea" prompted an exploratory study with regard to canine bacterial-diarrhea.[3] The P-A complex [marketed for pets as *PetFlora*[TM] Vitality Sciences Inc, Oakland Park, FL] was administered (250mg BID) to 10 dogs suffering from bacterial diarrhea during a kennel outbreak. In response to this outbreak, kennel areas and animals were first thoroughly cleansed and *all* animals were immediately administered PetFlora[TM] (as a prophylactic for those not showing symptoms). It is noteworthy that both food and water were made available to all – past experience suggesting that diarrhea could be readily controlled without restrictions. No signs of diarrhea were seen after 12 hours observation – this was certainly less-than the median of the 24-to-48 hours typical with a traditional antibiotic treatment (Neomycin generic "Biosol", 1.1cc/10kg, with food and possibility water restrictions). This [*PetFlora*[TM] vs. antibiotic] difference in diarrhea-duration of was very-highly significant ($P<0.002$, 2-tail, *Binomial Sign-Test*).[3, 6]

Supporting these "antibiotic-like actions" were observations of complete remission of IBS symptoms at one-year follow-up of patients maintained open-label for a 2 to 4 weeks period immediately following a double-blind study (4-6 weeks total).[2] Continuing remissions were observed in 62.5% in a group – at the 1-year follow-up – without further support (5/8), and in 100% of those (6/6) choosing maintenance P-A treatment [ultimately at reduced dosing, e.g., one cap every 1-3 days]. The final group of 10 patients – to generally good effect – chose intermittent use of P-A only when signs of IBS symptoms began to reappear.[2]

The body of past studies altogether encouraged our initiation of clinical studies of bacterial-diarrhea in populations at risk – the present study is represents a first step in this direction.

PURPOSE

The primary goal of this study was to evaluate clinical efficacy of *Prescript-Assist*[TM] (P-A), an advanced probiotic-prebiotic formulation for treatment of human-diarrhea in two population centers in Ecuador. A secondary goal was to explore the multivariate nature of the presenting diarrhea symptoms – particularly toward selecting measure(s) of disease severity and efficacy.

---

[2] No evidence of adverse-reactions or side-effects were reported either during either the formal study or at one-year follow-up.[1,2]

METHOD AND RESULTS

The body of this section first delineates methodological aspects of the study: *Participants and Test-Instrument*. This is followed by a joint consideration of analytic methods and their principal findings. This sets the stage for the final section – Discussion and Conclusions.

PARTICIPANTS

The study population was comprised of 21 patients (12♂ and 9♀) – presenting with persistent bacterial-diarrhea symptoms – almost equally drawn from two agrarian mountain communities located in mountainous regions about Quito, EC. *Miraflores*, served by Dra. Caicedo during the research study, is located 2.5 hours South of Quito; whereas, *Malchinqui*, about 1.25 hours North toward Cayambe, was served by Dr. De la Torre. Both communities – not surprising given continuing waves of diarrhea – were found to have bacterially contaminated public or well-water sources (e.g., *Fecal Coliforms*).[3] Patients – reflecting the largely *indios-mestizo* ethnicities of their communities – ranged in age between 2 to 65 years.[4]

TEST-INSTRUMENT

Recorded for each participant were: *Name, Age, Community, Sex* (♂ or ♀), and *Physician Observations/Comments*. Six primary symptoms also were assessed on a daily basis: *Diarrhea, Gases, Abdominal pain, Constipation, Vomiting*, and *Fever*. For research purposes, these symptoms were scored according to the number of days they were observed – starting with "1" at day of clinical diagnosis. Breaks – in any symptom – were conservatively scored as if present, if the symptom subsequently returned during the observational period. Using this approach each of the six symptoms was scored for *total days duration*.

ANALYSES AND FINDINGS

Analyses were conducted in three phases. During the Phase I, a *Principal Factor Analysis* (PFA) was conducted of the six clinical symptoms in a patients receiving P-A Treatment.[7,1] This provided for an exploratory analysis of dimensional "syndromic-factor" structure of the symptoms – akin to that reported in our earlier study of IBS.[1] In keeping with this earlier study, Analyses-of-Variance (ANOVAs) were planned for applications to any emergent sub-syndromic factors (with a focus on the main effects of Place-Community, Age, and Sex).[8,1,2] During Phase II, ANOVAs were conducted to evaluate the effects of Place (community), Sex, Age and selected interactions on the *log-transformed duration-of-diarrhea: Ln(D)*. Phase III follows this with final analyses comparing the log-transformed durations-of-diarrhea with P-A vs. community-specific experiences with standard antibiotic treatments.

---

[3]Contaminated food(s), perhaps not unrelated to water issues, were occasionally mentioned as the source of illness/diarrhea in some patient reports.

[4] SMI's IRB had approved the study protocol, which provided for incrementally extending treatment of outside the initial 5-65 year age-limits – if/as clinical experience supported efficacy and safety of P-A. No patients <2 years were treated for diarrhea during the study – this was reportedly was due to: the relative absence of the disease in infants (purportedly due to their being breast-fed till 2 years-of-age).

Phase I Analysis Findings

PFA revealed two factors that accounted for 68.8% of the total symptom variation. Table 1 presents the rotated factor matrix where it may be seen that the first factor "F1-Diarrhea-Vomiting" is essentially defined by loadings on *Diarrhea*(0.83) and *Vomiting* (0.88) with lesser though significant contributions by *Fever* (0.62*)* and *Nausea* (0.52). The second factor "Gas/Abdominal-Pain" is defined by almost identical loadings on these symptoms: *Gas* (0.92)*, Abdominal-Pain* (0.92) with no significant contributions by other variables.

Table 1. Rotated Factor Matrix*

FACTORS

SYMPTOMS	F1	F2
Diarrhea	0.828	-.352
Vomiting	0.884	-.095
Fever	0.620	0.221
Nausea	0.524	-.228
Gases	0.039	0.919
Abdominal Pain	-.288	0.918

*PFA with Varimax-Rotation.[7]

Table 2 summarizes the individual variable results of an analysis evaluating potential relationships with the first factor variable: *F1-Diarrhea-Vomiting*. Examining this table, a very highly significant difference may be seen to be associated with Place ($t(17)$ = 6.07, $P < 10^{-5}$ 2-tailed) – indicating that disease severity differed between the two communities. There is also a marginal indication ($P < 0.05$. 1-tailed) that disease (*Diarrhea-Vomiting*) is more severe in younger patients (*AgeDel = Age–24.4*). This suggestion also has a parallel in the analysis of the second factor (Gas/Abdominal-Pain) which appears ($t(17)$ = -1.80; $P < 0.05$, 1-tailed) to be most severe in younger patients (no other terms approach 0.05-significance nor did the overall model, $R^2(3, 17)$ =.213, P =0.24). These results altogether point to an essentially unitary disease, largely defined by Diarrhea-Vomiting and associated with marked community differences in intensity.

Table 2. ANOVA Model Summary for F1-Diarrhea-Vomiting*

MODEL-COEFFICIENTS

VARIABLE	B-Wt (Unstd. Coeff.)	STD. ERROR	BETA (Std. Coeff.)	t STATISTIC	SIGNIFICANCE LEVEL (P)
Place	0.744	0.123	0.762	6.067	$<10^{-5}$
AgeDel	-.012	0.006	0-.223	-1.827	0.085**
Sex	0.178	0.124	0.180	1.432	NS

*$R^2(3, 17)$ = 0.749 ($P < 2.4 \cdot 10^{-5}$)   ** $P<.05$ 1-tailed.

Phase II Analysis Findings

ANOVAs were initially conducted to first evaluate the effects of Place (community), Sex, Age and selected interactions on the *log-transformed duration-of-diarrhea: Ln(D)*. Results of this analysis were very highly significant ($R^2(5,14) = 0.868$, $P=10^{-5}$). Table 3 summaries the individual variable results, where it may be seen that the most prominent effects are associated with *Place* ($t(14) = 8.10$, $P <10^{-6}$) and its age-related interaction *"PxA"* ($t(14) = -2.31$, $P <0.02$). At the same time, the significant *SxA* interaction ($t(14) = 2.87$, $P <0.02$) points to a modulation of place result – depending on Sex and AgeDel. Evaluating these interactions in terms of "Days", it is clear that duration-of-diarrhea is less at the first community; 1.28 days for mean age (~25 years) patients across Sexes vs. 3.28 days in the second community.[5] This relative community advantage is somewhat increased in younger patients, but lessened as patients age (e.g., with 55 year-olds estimated as requiring 1.66 recovery days in the first community and only 2.55 days in the second).

Table 3. ANOVA Model Summary for Ln-Transformed Days [Ln (D)]*

MODEL-COEFFICIENTS

VARIABLE	B-Wt. (Unstd. Coeff.)	STD. ERROR	BETA (Std. Coeff.)	t STATISTIC	SIGNIFICANCE LEVEL (P)
Constant	0.722	0.059	–	–	–
Place (P)	0.474	0.058	0.814	8.10	$<10^{-6}$
AgeDel (A)	-.004	0.004	-.137	-1.12	NS
Sex (S)	0.061	0.060	0.103	1.43	NS
PxA	0.009	0.004	-.280	-2.31	<0.040
SxA	0.010	0.004	0.340	2.87	<0.013

*$R^2(5, 14) = 0.868$ ($P < 1.1 \cdot 10^{-5}$)

The *SxA* interaction also overlays the above cross gender-results suggesting some advantages for males, particularly before the end of adolescence (18 years). This appears to be increasingly offset by the tendency for males to experience longer bouts of diarrhea as they become older (increasingly so >25 years).

Phase III Analysis Findings

Compared in this final results section are the Log-transformed durations-of-diarrhea [Ln(D] with *P-A* vs. *"Past Antibiotic Experience."* Based on the medical experiences of the authors in their respective communities, diarrhea durations with traditional antibiotic treatment were estimated to be between respectively 48-72 hours and 72-96 hours (with either 7-day courses of *Amoxicillin or Ampicillin,* or the *Sulfamethoxazole-Trimethoprim* combination *Clotrimoxazol*).

---

[5]This requires the back (inverse) transformation of "log-transformed days" using the Exp-transformation. It should be noted that the back transformed days estimates would be maximum likelihood estimates (MLEs)– assuming analyses with Ln-Days resulted in MLE model coefficient estimates.

Comparison was first conducted for the community with an estimated 1.28 Days diarrhea-duration after P-A. Noting that 48-72 hours corresponds to diarrhea secession no-earlier-than Day 3, we conservatively choose to employ this as the standard for comparison [after appropriate Ln-transformations and Std-Errors drawn from Table 3). This comparison revealed a very highly significant statistical difference – with P-A treatment shortening diarrhea-duration to <43% of that experience with antibiotics ($t(14)$ = -10.28, $P < 10^{-7}$). Subsequently, a comparison was conducted for the community with an estimated 3.28 Days with P-A. Noting that 72-96 hours corresponds to secession no earlier than Day 4, we again conservatively tested with this as the standard for comparison (again with Ln-transformations and Std-Errors drawn from Table 3). This also revealed a significant difference – with P-A treatment shortening diarrhea-duration to <82% of that experience with antibiotics ($t(14) = -2.26$, $P < 0.04$).

Our final analysis was aimed at estimating the overall statistical significance of P-A vs. Antibiotic results by combining the significance levels from the two communities using the Pearson P_λ-Test.[8] This basic meta-analysis broadly supported our findings of significant reductions in the duration of diarrhea with *Prescript-Assist*^{TM} (P-A) vs. Antibiotics Treatment in Ecuador ($\chi 2(4) = 41.1$, $P < 2.6 \cdot 10^{-7}$).

DISCUSSION AND CONCLUSIONS

The primary goal of this study was to comparatively evaluate the clinical efficacy of *Prescript-Assist*[TM] (P-A), an advanced probiotic-prebiotic formulation for treatment of human-diarrhea in two communities in Ecuador. As seen in the previous section, diarrhea durations with traditional antibiotic treatment were estimated to be 48-72 hours and 72-96 hours in the respective study communities (with 7-day courses of either *Amoxicillin, Ampicillin,* or *Clotrimoxazol*). Comparisons against clinical experience – as in the present study – may be classed as a form of a *pre-post quasi-experimental research*.[9] Ordinarily, the *pre-post* design – particularly for single evaluative tests – is viewed as facing a number of potential validity challenges. These, however, may be largely offset by replications at different sites and in different populations – this in part motivated the two-community approach employed herein, and the earlier canine diarrhea study; as well as, our background presentation of supporting exploratory and formal clinical research.[3,1-2,4] The present *pre-post* study also may be strengthened by assuming a very conservative approach to establishing statistical significance – focusing on effects arguably too-large to be due to small validity challenges.[6] In the present study, *P-A vs. Antibiotic* comparisons for each community were constructed very conservatively, i.e., assuming the lower-bound of respective antibiotic treatment experiences [i.e., most rapid recovery]. Nonetheless, each of these comparisons proved statistically significant – with P-A associated with marked proportional reductions in duration in both communities (i.e., <43% to <86%). Overall statistical significance of the P-A vs. Antibiotic comparisons, computed across the individual communities, was found to be very-highly significant $[\chi2(4) = 41.1, \ P < 2.6 \cdot 10^{-7}]$. The body of findings – reflected herein and in earlier research – broadly supports the efficacy of *Prescript-Assist*[TM] (P-A) as a treatment for bacterial diarrhea.

A secondary goal – of the present study – was to explore the multivariate nature of the presenting diarrhea symptoms, particularly toward selecting measure(s) of disease severity and efficacy. As seen in the Phase I PFA results, some progress was made toward this end. Our findings essentially identified a unitary factor with significant loadings by all but *Gas* and *Abdominal-Pain* (which defined a second factor without much in the way of significant relationships with the experiment variables of interest). The dominant first factor "Diarrhea-Vomiting" was: (a) Found related to variables of interest; and (b) Broadly defined by loadings on *Diarrhea* (0.83) and *Vomiting* (0.88) with lesser though significant contributions by *Fever* (0.62*)* and *Nausea* (0.52). The prominent *Diarrhea* (0.83) loading – as well as its primary clinical significance – supported a focus on this variable during the analyses of Phase II.

Comparative efficacy and structural analysis goals of this study were largely met. However, as in all research, new opportunities and questions are suggested by the emergent findings. Our future interest will be toward more fully exploring the potential of advanced probiotic-prebiotic treatments for GI-track infections and conditions. The considerable promise seen in the present results certainly recommends clinical explorations of the emerging opportunities represented by *Prescript-Assist*[TM].

---

[6] This approach arguably compromises statistical power, but this is likely to not be an issue when effect sizes are very large – as anticipated in the present case from the earlier canine and clinical reports.

7

CONCLUSIONS

Three broad conclusions may be drawn from the body of reviewed and research findings presented in this report. These include:

- *Advanced probiotic-prebiotic combination "Prescript-Assist^{TM}"* has previously demonstrated efficacy against IBS and related gastric diseases in both short- and longer-term studies (e.g., 1-year follow-up).

- *Advanced probiotic-prebiotic "Prescript-Assist^{TM}"* demonstrated a comparative advantage – reduced duration – over some standard-antibiotics typically used to address bacterial diarrhea in humans.

- *Prescript-Assist^{TM}* – and other *advanced probiotic-prebiotic combinations* – have considerable promise as emerging treatments for a wide spectrum of acute and chronic GI diseases.

REFERENCES

1. Bittner, AC, Croffut, RM & Stranahan, MC (2005). Prescript-Assist^{TM} probiotic-prebiotic treatment for Irritable Bowel Syndrome: Randomized, placebo-controlled, double-blind clinical study. *Clinical Therapeutics, 27(6):755-761.*

2. Bittner, AC, Croffut, RM, Stranahan, MC & Yokelson, YN (2006). Prescript-Assist^{TM} Probiotic-Prebiotic Treatment for Irritable Bowel Syndrome (IBS): Post Cross-Over and One-Year Follow-Up Analyses. (Manuscript in preparation, Kent, WA: Bittner & Associates).

3. Bittner, AC & Smith, JM (2005). *Advanced Probiotic-Prebiotic Treatment for Canine Diarrhea (Report CS-02-05).* Ft. Benton, MT: Safer Medical, Inc.

4. Smith, C (2005). *Prescript-Assist™: Updated Synopsis of Clinical Experience (Report CS-01-05).* Ft. Benton, MT: Safer Medical, Inc.

5. NIH (2006). Pseudomembranous Colitis. In: *MedlinePlus Medical Encyclopedia* (Accessed 11 March 2006): http://www.nlm.nih.gov/medlineplus/ency/article/000259.htm

6. Gibbons, JD (1988). Sign Tests. In: *Encyclopedia of Statistical Sciences, Vol 8*:471-475. New York, NY: Wiley & Sons.

7. Harmon, H (1975). *Modern Factor Analysis (2nd ed).* Chicago, IL: University of Chicago Press.

8. Winer, BJ, Brown, DR & Michels, KM (1991). *Statistical Principles in Experimental Design (3rd ed).* San Francisco, CA: McGraw-Hill

9. Rossi, PH & Freeman, HE (1985). *Evaluation: A Systematic Approach. (3rd ed.)* Beverly Hills, CA: Sage.

Appendix - F: Special Rife Frequencies

Rife Frequencies

- **440 Hz:** Stimulates greater aggression, psycho social agitation, and emotional distres predisposing people to physical illness.
- **432 Hz:** Transmits beneficial healing energies because it is a pure tone of mathematics fundamental to nature.
- **400 - 480 Hz:** Destroys cancer cells.
- **444 Hz:** Kills cancer cells.
- **45 Hz:** Illness
- **30 Hz:** Marijuana Effect
- **6.66 Hz:** Depression/suicide
- **10.8 Hz:** Chaotic behavior
- **11 Hz:** Manic and riotous behavior
- **25 Hz:** Blindness if aimed at the head; heart attack if aimed at the chest.
- **147 Hz:** Reduces high blood pressure immediately.
- **153 Hz:** Relief of Muscular Dystrophy
- **174 Hz:** Pain relief
- **197 Hz:** Restores love of others, warmth (1 hour session)
- **528 Hz:** Repair DNA. Brings Positive Transformation I Solfeggio Sleep Music
- **447 Hz:** Relief Hemorrhoids, Crohns disease
- **417 Hz:** Wipes out all the Negative Energy
- **10000 Hz:** Full Restore TEETH Regeneration Regrowth Repair Frequencies; All 7 Chakras; 12 Meridians Chi Energy
- **456 Hz:** Head cold, Sinus infection
- **466 Hz:** Cancer glioblastoma tremor, Condylomata, venereal warts, papilloma virus.
- **852 Hz:** LET GO of Fear, Overthinking & Worries I Cleanse Destructive Energy I Awakening Intuition
- **5Hz, 26Hz, 79Hz, 80Hz, and 82:** For pain.
- **7Hz, 70Hz, 85Hz:** Acute pain.
- **76Hz:** For chronic pain.
- **7Hz, 66Hz:** Rheumatoid Arthritis.
- **11Hz, 17Hz, 53Hz, 55Hz, and 71Hz:** Emotional issues.
- **76Hz - 14Hz (sweep), 41Hz, and 70Hz:** Paralysis.
- **111Hz:** Tx 40 minutes a day for 5 days; brain starts to produce neurotransmitters; 3 to 5 days goes to normal and totally restores short term memory.
- **2.7KHz:** limb regrows.
- **90Hz sweep 111Hz:** stimulates beta endorphins.
- **4Hz:** stimulates catacolamines.
- **7.83Hz:** Schumann Resonance (frequency the earth vibrates.

Many of us spend our life time chasing mental images rather than observing the realities of life.

Appendix - G: Evidence for Intestinal Toxemia - An Inescapable Clinical Phenomenon

Evidence for intestinal toxemia— An inescapable clinical phenomenon

Alan Immerman, BS
Lombard, Illinois

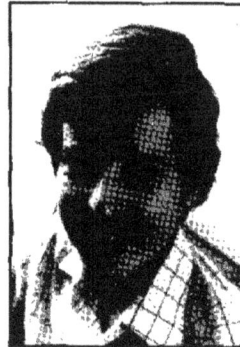

Alan Immerman

INTESTINAL TOXEMIA

A diet high in protein causes predominance in the intestine of proteolytic putrefactive bacteria which produce highly toxic compounds, some of which are absorbed. These compounds are incompletely detoxified by the liver, and therefore enter the systemic circulation. The toxins cause or aggravate many disease states. Alleviation of pathology can be accomplished by use of such non-traumatic measures as exercise, fasting, and proper diet. Intoxication arising from the intestine is a common occurrence and, if eliminated, health status may be expected to improve. Many aspects of the concept of intestinal toxemia are discussed.

Introduction

This paper will focus on the concept of intoxication of intestinal origin. The subject is of wide-ranging clinical importance and should be emphasized. As will be made clear, intestinal toxemia is frequently found as either a basic cause of or contributing factor to many clinical phenomena. In 1933, Dr Anthony Bassler, a professor of Gastroenterology at Fordham University Medical College and New York Polyclinic Medical College, and consulting gastroenterologist of Christs, Polyclinic and Peoples Hospitals in New York, stated, after a 25-year study of over 5000 cases, that: "Every physician should realize that the intestinal toxemias are the most important primary and contributing causes of many disorders and diseases of the human body."[1] Dr H.H. Boeker, in 1928, went so far as to say, "it is now universally conceded that autointoxication is the underlying cause of an exceptionally large group of symptom complexes."[2]

Intestinal toxemia is a process resulting from a certain type of diet or from intestinal obstruction. Various toxic chemicals are produced in the lumen by

Alan Immerman is presently enrolled in the National College of Chiropractic in Lombard, Illinois, where he is an honor student. He graduated in 1977 from Northern Arizona University, Magna Cum Laude with a BS in Chemistry, and was elected to the Phi Kappa Phi Honor Society. After graduation from chiropractic college in 1980, Immerman plans to practice in Phoenix, Arizona. His current address is Box 138, 200 E. Roosevelt Road, Lombard, Illinois 60148.

bacteria. These toxins are absorbed into the bloodstream either as a result of a pathological or a nonpathological state of the mucosa. Some of the toxins escape the detoxifying action of the liver because of pathological, functional (cannot act upon all of the toxin present), or physiological (normally does not act upon this toxin) liver insufficiency. These chemical poisons then enter the general circulation and exert deleterious effects before being excreted by the kidneys. The result of the intoxication is to produce a pathological change in the tissues, or to aggravate a previously existing condition. Each of these steps will be considered.

A thorough review of the literature was undertaken in the preparation of this paper. **Index Medicus,** from the years 1879 to 1978, was checked under multiple listings; many medical texts were perused to find leads to articles; the **Citation Index** was also checked. The result of this search was to find that almost no clinically-oriented articles have been written in the English language about intestinal toxemia since the late 1950s. In fact, few papers have been published since 1940 which directly address this subject. It is for this reason that most of the clinically-oriented papers reviewed in this paper are dated from before 1940.

The reader may wonder why the theory of intestinal toxemia has not been discussed in recent times, and is not well known today. The fact is that a change in opinion over the years, not based on any new scientific research, has led to the abandoning of this idea by the medical profession. It is important to emphasize that this has not resulted from new scientific research proving the error of the theory of intestinal toxemia. It is well known that certain ideas fall into and out of favor as the years pass, regardless of their validity, which has been the present case. An analogy may be drawn from the theory of chiropractic which, despite its great clinical usefulness, has been repeatedly "discovered" then abandoned or forgotten since ancient times; D.D. Palmer was the most recent individual to revive this old healing practice and bring it to our attention.

Some of the articles cited in this paper were written over 50 years ago. Quite naturally, a question may arise in the reader's mind as to whether or not such research could be reliable, having been done so many years ago. The answer to this is unequivocally affirmative. Portions of this paper as well as a great wealth of scientific information available today were uncovered many years ago, and are still valid. Modern textbooks in microbiology and biochemistry discuss many of the facts presented in this paper as true information; one text in each area is cited herein to demonstrate this point. Although scientific technology was not as sophisticated in the 1920s, the scientific intellect was equally keen; many important discoveries were made and theories confirmed. It is most important to emphasize that older research and

clinical observations are not necessarily invalid because of age.

The writer is well aware of the fact that current opinion in the medical world does not agree with the conclusions reached in this paper. However, the theory of intestinal toxemia as presented is scientifically and clinically sound; this ultimately is the main concern of an objective scientist. Opinion should be based on solid scientific research, and it is the purpose of this paper to aid in the formation of a scientifically-based opinion.

Effect of Diet

The experiments of Herter and Kendall[3], performed in 1909 at the Rockefeller Institute for Medical Research, were among the first to prove a definite connection between the nature of the diet and the type of bacterial flora found in the intestine. In experiments on cats (chosen because they are carnivores) and monkeys (chosen because of their biological similarity to man), it was proven that the intake of a high protein diet resulted in dominance of a strongly proteolyzing putrefactive type of flora (note: the term putrefaction refers to "decomposition of proteins by anaerobic organisms"[4]); also that conversion to a high carbohydrate/low protein diet resulted in dominance of a non-putrefactive type of flora. Fecal samples were cultured after a change in diet, and concentrations of endproducts of bacterial metabolism were measured in the urine to determine the type and character of the flora. The change in flora resulting from the change in diet was the same regardless of the animal type. The products of the putrefactive flora included indole and skatole (from tryptophan), phenol (from tyrosine), and hydrogen sulfide from the products of protein breakdown. Of importance to health care professionals is the following observation seen after a change in diet from high protein to high carbohydrate: "Clinically, the most striking feature of the change in diet [in monkeys] is an improvement in spirits and activity which may safely be construed as showing a markedly improved sense of bodily and psychological well being."[5] The results of these experiments were confirmed by other investigators of that same time period. [6,7,8,9] Many recent experiments have shown the presence of products in the urine of the putrefactive flora following ingestion of a high protein diet.[141,142,143,144,145,146,147,148] Other experiments have shown that ingestion of fermentable carbohydrates such as glucose, fructose or lactose results in delay of or complete inhibition of the putrefactive process.[141,148,149] Inhibition of the putrefactive process is reflected by decreased urinary output of putrefactive products.

Intestinal Obstruction

Obstruction in the intestine causes toxemia only in a small percentage of cases. However, it is far more likely to be rapidly fatal than toxemia resulting from diet. The main reason for considering obstruction is derived from the insight gained into the study of intestinal toxemia.

Obstruction in laboratory animals is produced by the surgical formation of a closed intestinal loop. The loop is washed to exclude the secretions of the stomach, liver, and pancreas, along with the products of food digestion. The result has been the same in all experiments; the bacteria multiply greatly, the proteolytic bacteria overgrow all others and produce toxic chemicals, the toxins are absorbed, and the animals become sick and die.[10,11,12,13,14,150] The toxins produced include histamine,[15] which is normally present but may be in a greater concentration, and various protein decomposition products.[16]

The toxins produced in the closed intestinal loop have been removed and injected into healthy animals with a reaction "more intense but similar to that developing in a closed-loop" animal.[17,18] Of importance is the fact that injection into the portal vein "gives a reaction similar to intravenous injection"[19] indicating that "the liver plays no essential role as a protective agent against this poison."[20]

These toxins have been produced by putrefactive bacteria which are normally present but have multiplied greatly and overgrown all other bacteria in the obstructed intestine. Therefore, it is within the realm of hypothesis that some amount of toxin is produced and absorbed in the case of intestinal stasis with a high intake of protein but without total obstruction.

It is important to emphasize again that intestinal obstruction similar to that observed in animals with surgical closure of an intestinal loop is rarely seen in man; such complete obstruction is certainly not the basic cause of intestinal toxemia, in most cases. However, insight into the process of intestinal toxemia probably can be gained by the consideration of such an extreme case; therefore, this consideration has been included. When researchers feed lab animals ten times the amount of saccharine a human being would ever consume in the same time period, identical logic is used. This logic is accepted by the scientific community. It is well recognized that much information can be gained from experiments with animals, using extreme conditions.

Nature and Action of Chemicals Produced by Proteolytic Bacteria

To date, the exact nature of all such chemicals has never been completely identified. Unfortunately, along with the development of instrumentation sophisticated enough to yield a complete answer to this question, there has been a simultaneous loss of interest in the subject of intestinal toxemia. However, much information is available from various research studies.

The reader should bear in mind a basic tenet of modern pathology which is too often forgotten today.

This tenet states that inflammation is a response of the body to tissue injury, and that this response serves to protect the body from the injurious agent.[151] Many times it is thought that the basic problem in a tissue involves inflammation, as if such a state existed in a vacuum. That would not be possible. Inflammation is the response of the body to local injury and attention should be paid to removal of the injurious agent, a truly protective response, rather than to suppressing the inflammation.

Some ammonia is formed by bacteria in the intestine, mainly from urea and digestive products of proteins[21]; ammonia is also formed, as is well known, by the liver and kidneys. In liver disease such as cirrhosis, or in disease of portal circulation, "abnormal elevations in the level of ammonia in peripheral blood may occur and these are accompanied by corresponding but lesser elevations of ammonia in the cerebrospinal fluid."[22] Many studies show that this increased concentration of ammonia causes severe neurological symptoms resembling hepatic coma such as mental disturbances, characteristic tremor, and altered EEG pattern.[23,24,25,26] A low protein diet minimized these symptoms.[23,24,26]

This reflects modern medical opinion as well. Harrison's **Principles of Internal Medicine** states that "both hepatic coma and the chronic form of hepatocerebral disease are characterized by hyperammonemia, which is probably important in their pathogenesis. Ammonium is derived from the bacterial action on intestinal proteins and normally is converted to urea in the liver.[152] Confusion, drowsiness, or other signs of impending hepatic coma should be treated by prompt decrease in protein intake to levels of 20 to 30 grams daily or less."[153] In regards to treatment for hepatic coma: "Reducing the protein intake, cleansing the colon of blood, suppressing the bacterial action on protein in the intestinal tract with neomycin or kanamycin, and administering the acidifying agent lactulose, all of which lower the NH_3 levels in the blood, have been found to restore many of these patients to a relatively normal state." And, "Although the biochemical mechanism is not fully understood, the most plausible hypothesis is that the levels of blood NH_3 are elevated because the diseased or bypassed liver fails to convert it to urea; the high serum NH_3 causes elevated NH_3 levels in the brain which interfere with its metabolism in some obscure way."[154] Ammonia may even be involved with the malignant transformation of cells.[27]

Clostridium perfringen enterotoxin has also been found.[28] This is well known to be highly poisonous.[29]

Indole is formed from tryptophan by proteolytic bacteria,[30] and is known to be toxic from results of experiments on animals,[31] and man.[32] It is also known that certain metabolites of tryptophan can cause bladder tumors.[33,34] With normal liver function, most, if not all indole is detoxified by the process of conjugation. In the case of sickness, this may or may not occur. A high protein, low carbohydrate diet results in increased excretion of conjugated indole, called indican,[7,35,141,146,147,148] as compared with a low protein, high carbohydrate diet. The amount of indican in the urine has been widely used as a measure of intestinal putrefaction.

However, indican determination used by itself is not reliable. For diagnostic purposes, it is interesting to know that combined determination of phenol and indican in the urine has proved to be highly valuable in the detection of the stagnant loop syndrome.[145] Stagnant loop syndrome is defined as bacterial overgrowth in the small intestine, vitamin B_{12} malabsorption, and steatorrhea, all of which improved by treatment with antibiotics.[155] This syndrome is believed to be present if the levels in the urine of both phenol and indican are abnormally elevated. Tabaqchali cautions, however, that since his experiment utilized only 51 patients, this observation of diagnostic reliability needs confirmation in a larger series.[145]

Phenol (carbolic acid) is formed from tyrosine in the process of putrefaction.[30,142,143,156] It is so extremely poisonous that it is used as an antimicrobial agent. It is both a local corrosive and systemic poison which can cause necrosis of gastrointestinal mucosa, renal and hepatic cells.[36] Phenol is absorbed into the body, and most of it is excreted in a free form — not conjugated and, therefore, not detoxified.[37,38] As is the case with indole, the concentration of phenol in the urine is increased with a high protein diet.[39,40,157,158]

Skatole is formed from bacterial action on tryptophan.[30,159] It is regarded as "a toxic substance causing depression of the circulation and of the central nervous system,"[32,41] and is found in increased concentration in the intestine following a high protein intake.[42] Skatole, "when in excess in the circulating blood through failure of conjugation by the liver," imparts a foul odor to the breath.[43] Skatole and indole are partially responsible for the characteristic odor of feces.[44] Skatole antagonizes acetylcholine and potassium[160] in smooth muscle preparations. Pseudomonas migula has recently been identified as a bacteria capable of converting tryptophan to skatole.[161] Following formation, skatole is converted into 6-hydroxyskatole by the cells of the gut wall, and possibly by other host tissues.[162] 6-hydroxyskatole damages lipid-absorbing cells, the hemoglobin within red blood cells, and hemoglobin found free within the body.[162] This destructive action probably accounts for the presence of metabolites of skatole in the urine of many patients suffering from the malabsorption syndrome and certain anemias.[162,164]

Hydrogen sulfide gas is another byproduct of protein decomposition.[43] In comparable concentrations it is "as toxic as cyanide and interferes with the cytochrome system."[45] It is obvious that this gas can irritate the mucosa; this brings about congestion and makes the mucosa more permeable to intestinal contents because of the presence of gas in solution. It may be responsible for "neurocirculatory myasthenic symptoms, for poisoning by this gas will cause: weakness, nausea, clammy skin, rapid pulse and cyanosis."[43]

Neurine is formed from sphingomyelin by anaerobic bacteria. This compound is toxic to animals.[46,47]

Aminoethyl mercaptan is formed from bacterial decomposition of the amino acid cysteine. It has a "profound hypotensive effect."[48]

Putrescine and cadavarine, formed from putrefaction of tryptophan, can lower blood pressure. Tryptamine, from the same source, raises blood pressure after an initial depression.[49]

Histamine is the last important decomposition product of tryptophan that is well known.[15,49,50] Poisoning with this compound can produce "headache, head congestion, nervous depression, cardiac arrythemia, fall of blood pressure, nausea, and collapse."[32]

Tyramine is a putrefactive product of tyrosine. It is structurally similar to epinephrine and can raise the blood pressure.[49,50]

It should be mentioned that some current writers hypothesize that putrefactive endproducts "irritate the receptor nerve-endings, thereby bombarding the associated spinal cord segments with afferent impulses, which result in muscular response and subluxations in the lower thoracic and upper lumbar areas, as well as predisposing to sacroiliac subluxation." Furthermore, "noxious materials in the bloodstream circulate to the central nervous system and . . . increase its irritability to afferent stimuli leading to increased hypertonicity of muscles and greater likelihood of subluxation."[51] We, therefore, may not have only the circulatory but also the nervous system mediating the effects of toxins to all the cells of the body.

Many other chemicals, too numerous to consider in detail, have been found to be formed in the intestine from bacterial putrefaction. These include guanidine,[52,53] and many others.[54,55] Besides the known substances, many chemicals of unknown character may be produced. Some of these chemicals may be toxic to a degree; of the toxins, some may be completely detoxified by the liver but others not at all. Other substances may be only partially rendered harmless. As is obvious, the subject of the chemistry of intestinal toxemia is highly complex and only partially understood. However, as will be seen, the situation from a clinical perspective is much clearer.

Intestinal Stasis

Delayed intestinal motility of the small and large intestines will now be discussed. Sir W. Arbuthnot Lane, MS, was one of the most knowledgeable men to work in this field. Being a surgeon, and having a penchant for surgical treatment of intestinal toxemia, he observed first hand the pathological state of the intestines of many sick people. His therapy, as might be suspected, was to remove the diseased section of the bowel; this was successful in providing temporary relief to the patient. However, as will be seen later, other treatments exist which are as successful but are non-traumatic and do not involve the use of drugs or surgery.

Lane defined chronic intestinal stasis as "an abnormal delay in the transmission of the intestinal contents through some portion or portions of the gastro-intestinal tract, which delay may be accompanied by constipation or by a daily or even more frequent action of the bowels."[56] He further states that any such delay facilitates multiplication of organisms and the subsequent development of toxemia in the bloodstream. This leads to "progressive degenerative changes in every tissue and a very definite and unmistakable series of symptoms."[56] It was mentioned in the discussion on intestinal obstruction that bacteria multiply greatly, with the proteolytic-putrefactive bacteria overgrowing all others. Is it not reasonable to consider that some of the features of chronic intestinal stasis are of the same kind but not as severe as those encountered in total obstruction?

Other physicians concur that delay (stasis) may be accompanied by one or more movements of the bowels per day.[57,58,59] This is of great clinical importance. It removes the foundation to the widely held belief that daily movements of the bowel are conducive to health.

Concerning clinical evidence, the following is worthy of mention. In a clinical study of 50 cases of intestinal toxemia, Dr H.J. Bartle found constipation in 72%, and delayed intestinal motility in 60%.[60] Dr Satterlee found constipation in 84% of his cases of intestinal toxemia[61]; in 1916, this doctor was attending physician to Fordham Hospital, Chief of Clinic for Gastroenterological Diseases, University and Bellevue Hospital Medical College, New York.

Consideration of the chemical aspect of intestinal stasis is also worthy of note. In this regard, Drs Underhill and Simpson of the department of Experimental Medicine, Yale University School of Medicine, state the following: "the effect of even mild constipation overshadows the effect of diet on the excretion of phenol and indican. Constipation causes a large increase in the excretion of these substances."[62]

In conclusion, it may be said that many physicians believed that delayed motility provides the foundation for building the condition of intestinal toxemia.[7,63,64,65,66,67]

Distension

Distension of the intestine has been attributed by some to be the cause of the symptoms of intestinal toxemia.[68] In experiments performed by Dr Alvarez of the Mayo Clinic, it was shown that pressure upon the rectum by sterile gauze could produce symptoms of intoxication.[69] There is no doubt that the effect of mechanical distension of the intestine is irritation to the nervous system, which is of no small importance. However, the presented evidence shows that mechanical irritation is indeed accompanied by chemical irritation. "Because it has been shown that constipation headache can occur in persons whose spinal cords have been cut, we know that this headache is not caused by nervous impulses from the colon. Therefore, it possibly results from absorbed toxic products or from changes in the circulatory system."[70]

Distension in obstruction of the intestine results in "more or less splanchnic congestion"[71] resulting in "interference with its [the mucosa] normal circulation."[72] This may result in functional or anatomic injury to the mucosa, allowing absorption of toxins to take place faster than the liver can detoxify them. Distension could lead to a "hemorrhagic and frequently necrotic condition of mucosa with a consequently hastened absorption of poisonous substances."[73]

As can be clearly seen, distension is a condition which the clinician will wish to reduce. Treatment will be discussed later.

Absorption

Absorption of toxins may occur through an intact gastrointestinal mucosa.[74,141] For example, a recent study has shown that indole and skatole can be rapidly absorbed at any level of the small or large intestine. In this experiment, medical students with normal health and patients in the hospital with no symptoms of gastrointestinal tract disease were used as subjects.[141] Many other writers feel that an inflammation of the mucosa is necessary before absorption will occur. Such inflammations of the rectosigmoid colon are described as "common."[75] Of 50 cases of intestinal toxemia examined by another physician, 80% had lower colon inflammation, and 62% had inflammation of the duodenum.[76] Others have reported general inflammation of the intestinal wall.[77,78] Inflammation of the terminal ileum or appendix will "elicit intense enterointestinal reflexes resulting in severe inhibition of gastrointestinal motility; as a result, functional obstruction often occurs in the small bowel."[79] Of interest is a description of the changes in the colon wall observed during the autopsy of insane patients residing at New Jersey State Hospital. Seen were large areas of destruction of mucosa plus atony and atrophy of smooth muscle.[80]

It is well known that mucosal injury may result in death from septicemia. Here it is stated that mucosal inflammation alters permeability, thereby allowing absorption of bacterial toxins which cause pathological changes in tissues. It is obvious that in septicemia, the bacteria produce metabolic toxins throughout the body. Many scientists believe these toxins are the cause of death in this type of situation.

Detoxification

Detoxification is primarily the responsibility of the liver. Though this subject has already been covered to a certain extent, a few additional remarks are necessary.

Detoxification is primarily the responsibility of the liver because the blood flowing from the stomach and intestines is "not returned directly from these organs to the heart, but is conveyed by the portal vein to the liver."[81] Once the portal vein has transported the blood to the liver, "this vein divides like an artery and ultimately ends in capillary-like vessels [sinusoids]."[81] From these sinusoids, substances absorbed from the intestines become exposed to liver parenchymal cells. These cells, hepatocytes, act upon such substances in many ways.

Ideally, hepatocytes will detoxify any poisons present and thereby protect the body. The important point here, however, is that toxins upon which the liver can act and detoxify, may be present in too great a quantity for complete liver action. As Dr Bartle says, the liver must be compared to other organs; "they can do just so much work and no more. In the case of the liver it is always carrying an unusual burden in chronic intoxication states, and naturally the breaking point must now and then be reached. This comes with an acute outburst of intoxicating symptoms. . . ."[82] With mucosal injury especially, "absorption of toxic substances may take place faster than the liver can detoxicate them and toxemia and death ensue."[73] Many authors concur in this viewpoint.[56,77] Of course, there are poisons against which "liver plays no essential role as a protective agent."[71] Phenol and skatole are examples of poisons which for the most part, escape liver action.[141,142,143,144,145,163]

Symptoms

Information on symptoms arising primarily from intestinal toxemia could fill volumes. Not only have books been written,[84] but literally thousands of articles in many languages have been published in the scientific literature on this topic. Obviously, an exhaustive discussion here is an impossibility.

No claim should be made that every symptom described in the following paragraphs arises from intestinal toxemia. However, by examination of the following, one must note that such toxemia is at the root of more problems than commonly imagined; it is at the root of many conditions more often than might be suspected.

Generally, intestinal toxemia manifests as one or more of the following: fatigue, nervousness, gastrointestinal conditions, impaired nutrition, skin manifestations, endocrine disturbances, neurocirculatory abnormalities and headaches.[43] Arthritis, sciatica and low back pain; allergy, asthma; eye, ear, nose and throat disease; cardiac irregularities; pathological changes in the breasts; all these conditions have responded to therapy directed at a toxemic state in the intestine, and the evidence for this follows. You will note that therapy is described only generally as being aimed at relieving the toxemic state of the intestine. To be more specific in each instance is impossible in this paper. Treatments mentioned will be representative of that which has been used by many doctors, not including surgery and drugs.

A. *Allergy:* Dr William Lintz, MD, successfully treated 472 patients suffering from "gastrointestinal allergy, a condition of hypersensitivity of the digestive tract," by eliminating the following allergens from the gastrointestinal tract: "bacteria and their toxins, foods and their split products."[85] The most frequent symptoms were endocrine gland disturbances of many types such as hypothyroidism, pituitary malfunction, etc; heart disease; hypertension, and many others.[86]

B. *Asthma:* Dr Allan Eustis, MD, instructor at Tulane University of Medicine in 1912, reports that 121 cases of bronchial asthma were relieved by eliminating the intestinal toxemia universally present.[87] Dr D. Rochester, MD, of the University of Buffalo School of Medicine in 1906, states that it is his conclusion, after 23 years of observation, that toxemia of gastrointestinal tract origin is the underlying cause of asthma. He says, "I believe the results of treatment justify my position."[88]

C. *Arthritis:* Dr Anthony Bassler treated 44 arthritic patients by relieving intestinal toxemia, and observed "marked improvement in 21, moderate in 19, none in four." With the addition of physical therapy, all but nine cases showed more marked improvement.[89] Twenty years later, Dr Bassler said a similar handling of 300 additional cases "has not modified my opinion a particle."[90] Sir W. Arbuthnot Lane, MS, FRCS (surgeon), believed that arthritis could not develop in the absence of intestinal toxemia, and says there is clinical and x-ray evidence of stasis in such patients. Furthermore, he states that, "the symptoms disappear and the patients recover sometimes with startling rapidity when the condition of stasis has been effectually dealt with."[91] Others confirm the connection between intestinal toxemia and arthritis.[92]

D. *Cardiac arrhythmias:* Guyton[93] states that "toxic conditions of the heart" can cause arrhythmias. Dr Bassler reports 100% success in eliminating such heart irregularities in 43 patients treated by reducing intestinal toxemia.[94] Dr Bainbridge, MD, stated that "intestinal toxemia is common among the causative factors of so-called functional heart disease.[95] Dr D.J. Barry in 1916, professor of Physiology, Queens College, Cork, England, stated that: "There seems little doubt that substances having a deleterious action on the heart musculature and nerves are formed both in the small and large intestine, even under apparently normal circumstances."[96]

Toxemia is further implicated in high blood pressure. Dr Hovell states that "toxemia due to intestinal sepsis is a common cause of increased blood pressure."[97]

E. *Ear, nose, and throat problems:* The experience of three doctors is neatly summed up by Dr J.A. Stucky, MD.[98] "In several hundreds of cases of diseases of the nasal accessory sinuses, middle and internal ear, ... I have found unmistakable and marked evidence of toxemia of intestinal origin as evidenced by excessive indican in the urine, and when the condition causing this was removed there was marked amelioration or entire relief of the disease."[99,100]

F. *Eclampsia:* R.C. Brown, MB, MS, FRCS, an obstetrical surgeon in England in 1930, linked intestinal toxemia and eclampsia.

G. *Eye problems:* Dr C.W. Hawley, MD, treated many cases of eye strain and disease with success once again by relieving intestinal toxemia.[101]

H. *Thyroid gland disease:* Dr W.S. Reveno, MD, theoretically links exophthalmic goiter to "a toxic process in the intestinal tract."[102] He cites animal studies as evidence. Echoing this view is Dr A. Eustis, MD, who cites case histories of patients who found complete relief from exophthalmic goiter as a result of eliminating intestinal toxemia.[103] Sir W.A. Lane reports a connection between intestinal toxemia and "several changes in the thyroid" such as "adenomatous growths."[104]

I. *Nervous system:* Many disorders of the nervous system are involved. Dr Carl Von Noorden, MD, professor of the First Medical Clinic, Vienna, Austria, in 1913, described a condition of diffuse sensory polyneuritis with pronounced vagal irritation, treated with positive results by relieving intestinal toxemia. He and his assistant extracted a "poisonous substance from the feces, which in animal experiments produced quite similar symptoms."[105] This substance was found to be formed by a "bacterium of the paratyphus group."[106]

Dr C.A. Herter, MD, in 1892, lecturer on Anatomy and Pathology of the Nervous System, New York Polyclinic, linked intestinal putrefaction to epilepsy in 31 patients. He based this on a successful treatment using drugs to control bacterial activity of the intestine.[107] Agreeing with his conclusion are other doctors.[108,109]

Drs Satterlee and Eldridge, in a paper read to the annual session of the American Medical Association in 1917, reported experience with 518 cases of "mental symptoms" including "mental sluggishness, dullness and stupidity; loss of concentration and/or memory; mental incoordination, irritability, lack of confidence, excessive and useless worry, exaggerated introspection, hypochondriasis and phobias, depression and melancholy, obsessions and delusions,

hallucinations, suicidal tendencies, delirium, and stupor."[110] Their success in eliminating these symptoms by surgically relieving intestinal toxemia is truly remarkable in the light of today's commonly-held beliefs. In the discussion following the presentation of the doctors' paper, other physicians stated that they shared in this experience.[111]

Other authors describe the same pattern, adding headache [66,91,109,112] to the list of symptoms. It would indeed appear true that "the nervous system is almost invariably affected in whole or in part by chronic intestinal toxemia" and that "the nervous symptoms are often the most prominent in the symptomatology."[111]

Of considerable interest is a recent paper entitled, "Biochemical Aspects of Indole Metabolism in Normal and Schizophrenic Subjects" by Herbert Sprince.[163] In this highly sophisticated paper, 11 independent laboratories are noted to have found at least five times more 6-hydroxyskatole in the urine of schizophrenics than in that of normal subjects. Such universal agreement, Sprince says, is highly significant since this is an area where conflict, not agreement, is the rule.[163] It will be remembered that 6-hydroxyskatole arises primarily from skatole in the intestine and that skatole arises from the action of putrefactive bacteria on tryptophan, an essential amino acid.

J. *Senility:* The following should be mentioned: "Auto-intoxication from intestinal stasis or from constipation due to lessened peristaltic activity, undoubtedly plays a contributing part in the process of senescence."[113]

K. *Low back pain and sciatica:* Dr R.B. Osgood, MD, cites six cases of patients suffering from these conditions. A few had also received chiropractic manipulative care with no improvement. In these cases, the cause was a toxemic state of the intestine; the pain completely left upon elimination of the toxemia, and returned upon a return of toxemia because of dietary errors. His references point to other physicians who had the same experience.[114]

In this regard, Dr Von Noorden found "pains especially frequent which corresponded to the ordinary sciatic or intercostal neuralgia."[115] The reader would be well advised to review the facts on irritation to the nerves of the low back area during a toxemic state of the intestine.

L. *Dermatoses:* Dr Hans J. Schwartz, MD, in a statistical analysis of 900 patients suffering from acne, eczema, and many other skin conditions, concluded that "intestinal toxemia is an important etiologic factor in the production of many dermatoses, especially those of the inflammatory type."[116] Dr J.F. Burgess, MB, lecturer in Dermatology, McGill University, associate dermatologist, Montreal General Hospital, reports the results of studying 109 cases of eczema. He states that "on the basis of clinical observations and sensitivity tests against various amino acids and ptomaine bases, eczema is probably caused by intestinal toxemia."[117] Others concur.[118,119]

M. *Breast pathology:* Changes in the breast resulting from intestinal toxemia have been described by many doctors. The views of three can be summarized as such[120]: "The breasts undergo degenerative changes, manifested in the first instance as induration, to be followed by inflammatory and cystic degeneration, and possibly, lastly, by cancerous infection."[95,121]

N. *Cancer:* There is no claim that intestinal toxemia is the cause of cancer. However, some physicians believe that "even the beginning of malignant disease of various organs comes within the wide range of intestinal stasis."[92] Sir W.A. Lane recorded his feeling of being "exceedingly impressed by the sequence of cancer and intestinal stasis."[122]

In light of the clonal selection theory of chemical carcinogenesis which states that "all chemical carcinogens will display . . . a greater toxicity for normal tissue cells than for the cells of a tumor derived therefrom by treatment with that carcinogen,"[123] it can be speculated that toxins of intestinal origin may initiate malignant transformations. The malignant cell would be more resistant to the toxic effects than would a normal cell, according to this theory.

Treatment

In the treatment of intestinal toxemia various measures have been used. These include surgical removal of inflamed, ulcerated, or infected intestine (sometimes including the entire colon); autogenous vaccines to kill the bacteria responsible for the production of the toxins; colonics and/or laxatives for obvious reasons; diet therapy, and exercise. Different doctors have used various combinations of these therapeutic measures; some have put great emphasis on surgery, while others none at all. Many have put emphasis on the use of vaccines to some degree. Some recommend colonics and/or laxatives; others literally condemn their use. Almost all have used some type of diet therapy, and exercise has often been recommended.

The author's conception of an ideal therapy will now be described. It is an amalgam of the ideas of the many clinicians cited in this paper, but with the addition of a few basic holistic concepts in the light of the axiom, "Physician, do no harm."

First, if vaccines and surgery can be avoided by the use of other less traumatic and less side-effect-producing therapies which are at least equally efficacious, then vaccines and surgery should not be used. This does not mean that drug and surgical therapies are never needed in the treatment of intestinal toxemia; however, these therapies are almost never needed.

Second, any therapeutic measure which provides only the relief of symptoms is inferior to a measure that removes the cause of the symptoms; symptomatic relief is only temporary, whereas, the removal of the cause leads to permanent relief. These concepts are probably self-evident and surely constitute common sense. Surely no chiropractic physician would argue with this general overview of treatment.

Since a majority of physicians have found success in the use of diet therapy and exercise, these measures will be emphasized. Diet therapy is non-traumatic, does not produce side-effects, and removes the cause of the toxemia. It allows for a complete cure to take place which lasts as long as the diet is followed. Dr Satterlee stated that "diet and proper emptying of the bowels has always been the recognized treatment."[124]

Treatment can be summarized by the following: "Patients must be taught how to eat, how to live, how to work and how to play. It must be impressed on them that health will not return through the simple act alone of taking medicine from a bottle. If they can be made to see that a general cleaning-up process is to be inaugurated, and that it is their duty to keep things cleaned up as treatment progresses, and after it is ended, and that the whole management of their trouble is really founded on very ordinary principles, then, with great interest, they usually cooperate quite heartily with their physician."[125]

If the reader will refer to the effect of diet on putrefaction, he will see that animal experiments indicate the benefit of a low protein, high carbohydrate diet. This concept is universally agreed upon by the physicians noted in this paper. How much protein should be consumed? The controversy over this issue is great. However, since "protein in an average food intake of 2,500 calories is about 94 grams per day"[126] and the recommended daily allowance is 50-60 grams for adults, it is obvious that an immediate decrease in intake by almost 50% can be safely accomplished. In light of studies on minimum protein requirements, we may even consider as sufficient intakes of 15-25 grams per day of high quality protein.[127] Obviously, with this intake of protein, other food components are to be relied upon to supply energy needs.

The remainder of the diet should contain a minimal amount of fat, with carbohydrates supplying the bulk of the energy need. It has been shown that fats, especially heated fats, intensify the process of intestinal toxemia.[128] The dietary carbohydrates should not be the refined or starchy form. The more easily digested and more highly nutritious types are preferred. Therefore, after the intestine has healed, fruits and vegetables should be used to provide the greatest amount of the carbohydrate intake, and thus the caloric requirement. These foods have the additional benefit of being rich in the vitamins and minerals.

Intake of certain specific items should be either greatly reduced or eliminated. These include sugar,[129] as implied above; salt, alcohol, condiments, tobacco[130]; tea, coffee, pastry, fried foods, and "any article of food which is known to disagree."[88]

Eating the correct amount of food is an essential feature of the proper diet. Dr Stucky, MD, says that "all forms of food, when eaten in greater quantities than the digestive fluids can digest, are capable of forming putrefactive poisons, which are deleterious to the human organism. I have, therefore, insisted that all my patients should eat small meals in which the protein foods should form a very small proportion."[131] Dr Rochester, MD, says "the amount of food should be limited to the minimum compatible with maintenance of health and weight."[88] Echoing this is Dr Synnott: "Patients do better and feel better when the caloric intake in their diet is curtailed."

In the acute stage, no food at all is recommended. "Feeding bulky foods causes further distension of the colon, an added burden is put upon its weakened walls, the damaged bowel musculature is taxed beyond the power to respond, the delayed motility and stasis are increased, the gastroptosis and enteroptosis are aggravated, the expected increase in peristalsis does not occur, but on the contrary there is more pronounced paresis of the already atonic, overworked and disabled bowel."[132] Dr Bartle concurs in this view.[130]

Instead of feeding, fasting is recommended. "Fasting is a perfectly sound method of diminishing toxins if combined with copious draughts of water."[133] Fasting has been shown to reduce the phenols to a low level.[134] It has also been shown to increase by one to two days to over two weeks the life span in dogs with duodenal obstruction; the dogs were forced to fast for four days prior to surgical creation of the obstruction.[135] In a 76 kilogram man, "intestinal putrefaction as measured by the output of urinary indican was markedly decreased during the fasting interval" of seven days.[136] Fasting will rest the overworked intestine and allow the physiological process of inflammation to proceed onward to the process of repair. One need not worry about starvation in these cases, since the patients already are suffering from excess food intake.

The administration of Lactobacillus acidophilus culture and lactose is said by some to be of great value; but others claim that they are useless. It is interesting to note that the entire basis for the idea that yogurt and its bacteria are beneficial to health is based on the theory of intestinal toxemia. The idea is that the "good bacteria" (Lactobacillus) will displace the "bad," namely the putrefactive proteolytic type. This therapy seems to have some value, at least in a percentage of cases. However, in light of its having dubious value in some doctors' opinion, this therapy should not be relied upon.

The topic of colonic irrigations is surrounded by much argument and controversy. There are some who claim that colonics have great therapeutic value,[137,138] and as might be suspected, others avoid its use and decry its value.[139] Dr Von Noorden states that such treatments "only hide the pathologic condition of the intestine. Instead of helping, they retard the definite cure. They are justified and advantageous only in acute disease."[105] Dr Bassler says that colonics "relieve the toxemia by clearing the large bowel for a few days but do nothing to control the bacteriology or the chemistry . . . since the locality for most of the toxic process is in the small intestine. Kept up long enough, they do more harm than good."[140]

Surrounding the subject of exercise there is no controversy, just ignorance or advocacy. Of those in favor, Dr Bassler presents an average view. "Physical exercise, especially in the open, is valuable to keep back the assault of toxins on body tissues. This is accomplished by increasing the conjugating ability by calling forth higher degrees of protoplasmic activity, higher oxidation and increased circulation."[57] But the clinician should be wary, since increased circulation may carry toxins to previously unexposed tissues, thereby multiplying the symptoms. As is usual in the health care profession, prudent clinical judgment is in order.

If the outlined program is followed, both the doctor and patient will be satisfied with the results.

Discussion

Toxemia and subsequent pathology may result from absorption of certain chemicals formed by bacterial action on amino acids. Pathology is classically defined as abnormal function. The sources mentioned in the section on *symptoms* reveal that there is a clinical, clearly observable relationship between intestinal toxemia and abnormal cellular function. These studies report thousands of cases of people suffering from various ills who became well after clearing up their intestinal toxemia. For example, eczema is a pathological change; it healed time and again when the source of irritation, intestinal toxemia, was removed. The author is aware that this is a controversial idea, today. But, nonetheless, it is certainly conceivable that, for example, the following sequence could occur: high protein diet results in phenol (corrosive poison) production; phenol enters circulation, causing local pathology. Evidence has been presented that a high protein diet causes proliferation of proteolytic bacteria; it is well known that such proteolytic bacteria produce phenol from the amino acid tyrosine, and that phenol can kill cells; papers have been reviewed that prove that the majority of absorbed phenol is not conjugated by the liver, and therefore not detoxified; and many papers have been reviewed which relate pathology to the presence of intestinal toxemia in a statistically significant way.

For example, when previously discussing *dermatoses*: 1017 patients were examined and treated. In a clinical discussion, it is highly relevant and important that many sick people become well when their intestinal toxemia is cleared up. On the other hand, medical opinion states that the etiology of such diseases as Crohn's, Whipple's, ulcerative colitis, and many others, is unknown (idiopathic). But the irritation that causes the primary inflammation in these afflictions must come from somewhere, or the entire science of pathology is in error. It has been proposed in this paper that the products of intestinal putrefaction are a significant source of such irritation.

Summary and Conclusions

The following have been stated:

1) Change in diet induces change in intestinal flora. With a high protein diet, proteolytic putrefactive bacteria predominate.

2) Such bacteria produce highly toxic compounds, some of which are absorbed.

3) The liver does not detoxify all of these toxins; thus, some escape into the general circulation and can be found in the urine.

4) These toxins produce a wide range of symptoms and aggravate preexisting pathologies.

5) The problems resulting from such an intoxication may be eliminated in almost all cases by a judicious combination of fasting, exercise, and proper diet consisting of small amounts of protein and fat with enough carbohydrates to supply the caloric need. The best carbohydrates are in fruits and vegetables.

6) Intestinal toxemia is frequently found to be either the basic cause of or contributing factor to many clinical phenomena, and the holistic practitioner is advised to bear this in mind. □

References

1. Bassler, A.: "Intestinal Toxemia," *Medical Journal and Record*, Vol 136, 1933, p 322.
2. Boeker, H.H.: "Autointoxication," *Medical Journal and Record*, Vol 128, Sept 19, 1928, p 293.
3. Herter, C.A. and Kendall, A.I.: "The Influence of Dietary Alterations on the Types of Intestinal Flora," *Journal of Biological Chemistry*, Vol 7, 1909-10, pp 203-235.
4. Orten, J.M. and Newhaus, O.W.: *Human Biochemistry*, 9th ed, C. V. Mosby Company, St Louis, Missouri, 1975, p 469.
5. Herter, *op cit*, p 216.
6. Cannon, P.R., Dragstedt, L.R., and Dragstedt, C.A.: "Intestinal Obstruction," *Journal of Infectious Disease*, Vol 27, 1920, pp 139-144.
7. Underhill, F.P. and Simpson, G.E.: "The Effect of Diet on the Excretion of Indican and the Phenols," *Journal of Biological Chemistry*, Vol 44, 1920, pp 69-97.
8. Torrey, J.C.: "The Regulation of the Intestinal Flora of Dogs through Diet, "*Journal of Medical Research*, Vol 39, 1918-19, pp 415-447.
9. Folin, O. and Denis, W.: "The Excretion of Free and Conjugated Phenols and Phenol Derivatives," *Journal of Biological Chemistry*, Vol 22, 1915, p 309.
10. Gerard, R.W.: "Chemical Studies on Intestinal Intoxication," *Journal of Biological Chemistry*, Vol 52, 1922, pp 111-124.
11. Cannon, *op cit*, pp 139-144.
12. Stone, H.B., Bernheim, B.M., and Whipple, G.H.: "Intestinal Obstruction: A Study of the Toxic Factors," *Bulletin of The Johns Hopkins Hospital*, Vol 23, No 256, 1912, pp 159-165.
13. Gerard, R.W.: "The Lethal Agent in Acute Intestinal Obstruction," *Journal of the American Medical Association*, Vol 79, No 19, 1922, pp 1581-1584.
14. Whipple, G.H., Stone, H.B., and Bernheim, B.M.: "Intestinal Obstruction," *Journal of Experimental Medicine*, Vol 17, 1913, pp 286-307.
15. Gerard, R.W.: "Chemical Studies on Intestinal Intoxication," *Journal of Biological Chemistry*, Vol 52, 1922, pp 111-124.
16. Gerard, R.W.: "The Lethal Agent in Acute Intestinal Obstruction," *Journal of the American Medical Association*, Vol 79, No 19, 1922, pp 1581-1584.
17. Stone, H.B., Bernheim, B.M., and Whipple, G.H.: "Intestinal Obstruction: A Study of the Toxic Factors," *Bulletin of The Johns Hopkins Hospital*, Vol 23, No 256, 1912, pp 159-165.
18. Whipple, G.H., Stone, H.B., and Bernheim, B.M.: "Intestinal Obstruction," *Journal of Experimental Medicine*, Vol 17, 1913, pp 286-307.
19. Whipple, *ibid*, p 306.
20. Whipple, *ibid*, p 305.
21. Wilson, D.R., Ing, T.S., Metcalfe-Gibson, A., and Wrong, O.M.: "**In Vivo** Dialysis of Faeces as a Method of Stool Analysis. III. The Effect of Intestinal Antibiotics," *Journal of Clinical Science*, Vol 34, 1968, pp 211-221.
22. McDermott Jr, W.V., Adams, R.D., and Riddell, A.G.: "Ammonia Levels in Blood and Cerebrospinal Fluid," *Proceedings of Society of Experimental Biology and Medicine*, Vol 88, 1955, p 382.
23. McDermott, W., Adams, R.D.: "Eck-Fistula — A Cause of Episodic Stupor in Humans," *Journal of Clinical Investigation*, Vol 32, 1953, pp 587-588.
24. Phillips, G.B., Schwartz, R., Gabuzda, G.J., and Davidson, C.S.: "The Syndrome of Impending Hepatic Coma in Patients with Cirrhosis of the Liver Given Certain Nitrogenous Substances," *The New England Journal of Medicine*, Vol 247, No 7, 1952, pp 239-246.
25. Berger, R.L., Liversage, R.M., Chalmers, T.C., Graham, J.H., McGoldrick, D.M., and Stohlman Jr, F.S.: "Exchange Transfusion in the Treatment of Fulminating Hepatitis," *The New England Journal of Medicine*, Vol 274, No 9, 1966, pp 497-499.
26. Sherlock, S., Summerskill, W.H.J., White, L.P., Phear, E.A.: "Portal-Systemic Encephalopathy. Neurological Complications of Liver Disease," *The Lancet*, Vol 2, Sept 4, 1954, pp 453-457.
27. Visek, W.J., Kolodny, G.M., and Gross, P.R.: "Ammonia Effects in Cultures of Normal and Transformed 3T3 Cells," *Journal of Cell Physiology*, Vol 80, 1972, pp 373-382.
28. Williams, B.W.: "Importance of Toxemia Due to Anaerobic Organisms in Acute Intestinal Obstruction and Peritonitis," *The Lancet*, Vol 1, April 30, 1927, pp 907-912.
29. Jawetz, E., Melnick, J.L., Adelberg, E.A.: *Review of Medical Microbiology*, 12th ed, Lange Medical Publications, Los Altos, California, 1976, pp 189-190.
30. Orten, *op cit*, p 471.
31. Herter, C.A.: "An Experimental Study of the Toxic Properties of Indol," *NY Medical Journal*, Vol 68, July 16, 1898, pp 89-93.
32. Korenchevsky, V.: "Autointoxications and Processes of Aging," *Texas Rep Biology and Medicine*, Vol 12, 1956, p 1016.
33. Bryan, G.T., Brown, R.R., and Price, J.M.: "Incidence of Mouse Bladder Tumors Following Implantation of Paraffin Pellets Containing Certain Tryptophan Metabolites," *Cancer Research*, Vol 24, 1964, pp 582-585.
34. Kerr, W.K., Barkin, M., Levers, P.E., Woo, S.K-C, and Menczyk, Z.: "The Effect of Cigarette Smoking on Bladder Carcinogens in Man," *The Canadian Medical Association Journal*, Vol 93, No 1, 1965, pp 1-7.
35. Herter, *op cit*, pp 203-235.
36. Robbins, S.L.: *Pathologic Basis of Disease*, 1st ed, W.B. Saunders Company, Philadelphia, 1974, p 520.
37. Folin, *op cit*, p 320.

38. Dubin, H.: "Physiology of the Phenols," *Journal of Biological Chemistry*, Vol 26, 1916, p 99.
39. Folin, *op cit*, p 317.
40. Underhill, *op cit*, p 96.
41. Salant, W. and Kleitman, N.: "The Toxicity of Skatol," *Journal of Pharmacology and Experimental Therapeutics*, Vol 19, 1922, p 313.
42. Herter, *op cit*, p 215.
43. Bartle, H.J.: "Protein Intoxication," *Medical Journal and Record*, Vol 128, July 4, 1928, p 30.
44. Orten, *op cit*, p 335.
45. Challenger, F. and Walshe, J.M.: "Foeter Hepaticus," *The Lancet*, Vol 1, 1955, p 1240.
46. Orten, *op cit*, p 467.
47. Haubold, H.A.: "General Considerations Regarding Self-Intoxication," *The NY Medical Journal*, Vol 60, Dec 25, 1897, p 857.
48. Orten, *op cit*, p 468.
49. Orten, *ibid*, p 472.
50. Baker, C.E.: "The Physiological Effects of Certain Toxic Substances of Gastro-Intestinal Origin," *Illinois Medical Journal*, Vol 51, April 1927, pp 325-327.
51. Homewood, A.E.: *The Neurodynamics of the Vertebral Subluxation*, 3rd ed, Valkyrie Press, St Petersburg, Florida, 1977, pp 77-78.
52. Korenchevsky, *op cit*, p 1815.
53. Major, R.H.: "Relationship Between Certain Products of Metabolism and Arterial Hypertension," *Journal of the American Medical Association*, Vol 83, No 2, 1924, pp 81-84.
54. Barger, G. and Dale, H.H.: "Chemical Structure and Sympathomimetic Action of Amines," *Journal of Physiological Chemistry*, Vol 41, 1910-1911, pp 19-59.
55. Korenchevsky, *op cit*, pp 1006-1036.
56. Lane, W.A.: "Chronic Intestinal Stasis," *Journal of Surgery, Gynecology and Obstetrics*, Vol 16, 1913, p 600.
57. Bassler, A.: "Chronic Intestinal Toxemia," *Medical Record*, Vol 145, 1937, p 160.
58. Hertz, A.H.: "Chronic Intestinal Stasis," *The British Medical Journal*, Vol 1, April 19, 1913, p 817.
59. Binnie, J.F.: "Symptoms of Colonic Intoxication," *Journal of American Medical Association*, Vol 58, No 26, 1912, p 2011.
60. Bartle, *op cit*, p 63.
61. Satterlee, G.R.: "Chronic Intestinal Stasis," *American Journal of Medical Science*, Vol 152, 1916, p 729.
62. Underhill, *op cit*, p 96.
63. Lane, *op cit*, pp 600-606.
64. Satterlee, *op cit*, pp 727-738.
65. Hertz, *op cit*, pp 817-821.
66. Lucas, C.G.: "Symptomatology of Chronic Intestinal Stasis," *Southern Medical Journal*, Vol 17, No 9, 1924, pp 659-661.
67. Bartle, *op cit*, pp 63-66.
68. Tucker, John: "Intestinal Toxemia," *Medical Clinics of North America*, Vol 19, May 1936, pp 1819-1830.
69. Alverez, W.C.: *An Introduction to Gastro-enterology*, 4th ed, Paul B. Hoeber, Inc, New York; NY, 1948, p 638.
70. Guyton, A.C.: *Textbook of Medical Physiology*, 5th ed, W.B. Saunders Company, Philadelphia, 1976, p 674.
71. Whipple, G.H., Stone, H.B., and Bernheim, B.M.: "Intestinal Obstruction," *Journal of Experimental Medicine*, Vol 17, 1913, p 305.
72. Gerard, R.W.: "The Lethal Agent in Acute Intestinal Obstruction," *Journal of the American Medical Association*, Vol 79, No 19, 1922, p 1583.
73. Cannon, *op cit*, p 143.
74. Whipple, G.H., Stone, H.B., and Bernheim, B.M.: "Intestinal Obstruction," *Journal of Experimental Medicine*, Vol 17, 1913, p 322.
75. Soper, H.W.: "The Mucosa of the Rectum and Sigmoid Colon as a Focus of Infection," *Boston Medical and Surgical Journal*, Vol 176, No 22, 1917, p 766.
76. Bartle, *op cit*, p 64.
77. Lucas, *op cit*, p 660.
78. Woolley, P.G.: "Intestinal Stasis and Intestinal Intoxications: A Critical Review," *Journal of Laboratory and Clinical Medicine*, Vol 1, 1915-1916, p 50.
79. Guyton, *op cit*, p 897.
80. Synnott, M.J.: "Intestinal Toxemia, Its Diagnosis and Treatment," *Medical Journal and Record*, Vol 136, No 11, 1932, p 441.
81. Warwick, R. and Williams, P.L.: *Gray's Anatomy*, 35th British ed, W.B. Saunders Company, Philadelphia, 1973, p 588.
82. Bartle, *op cit*, p 387.
83. Haubold, *op cit*, p 859.
84. Bassler, A.: *Intestinal Toxemia Biologically Considered*, F.A. Davis Company, Philadelphia, 1930.
85. Lintz, W.L.: "Gastrointestinal Allergy," *The Review of Gastroenterology*, Vol 6, 1939, p 321.
86. Lintz, *ibid*, pp 320-332.
87. Eustis, A.: "Further Evidence in Support of the Toxic Pathogenesis of Bronchial Asthma, Based upon Experimental Research," *American Journal of Medical Science*, Vol 143, 1912, p 863.
88. Rochester, D.: "The Treatment of Asthma," *Journal of the American Medical Association*, Vol 47, No 24, 1906, p 1984.
89. Bassler, A.: "The Colon in Connection with Chronic Arthritis (Arthritis Deformans)," *American Journal of Medical Science*, Vol 160, 1920, p 357.
90. Bassler, A.: "Aging, Arteriosclerosis, and Cardiac Conditions," *Medical Record*, Vol 153, Jan 1, 1941, p 21.
91. Lane, W.A.: "Consequences and Treatment From a Surgical Point of View," *British Medical Journal*, Vol 1, March 15, 1913, p 547.
92. Lucas, *op cit*, p 661.
93. Guyton, *op cit*, p 213.
94. Bassler, A.: "Coronary Disease and the Intestine," *Medical Record*, Vol 155, April 1, 1942, p 249.
95. Bainbridge, W.S.: "The Constitutional Effect of Prolonged Intestinal Toxemia," *Medical Journal and Record*, Vol 122, No 8, 1925, p 438.
96. Barry, D.T.: "Intestinal Toxins and the Circulation," *The Lancet*, Vol 2, July 1, 1916, p 15.
97. Hovell, T.M.: "Gastro-intestinal Sepsis, a Cause of Meniere's Symptoms," *Proceedings of the Royal Society of Medicine*, Vol 11, No 3, 1918, p 16.
98. Stucky, J.A.: "Intestinal Autointoxication as a Factor in the Causation of Pathologic Conditions of the Ear, Nose and Throat," *Journal of the American Medical Association*, Vol 53, No 15, 1909, p 1185.
99. Hovell, *op cit*, pp 15-18.
100. Gatewood, W.L.: "Symptoms of Gastrointestinal Origin in the Ear, Nose and Throat," *Archives of Otolaryngology*, Vol 33, 1941, pp 592-598.
101. Hawley, C.W.: "Autointoxication and Eye Diseases," *Ophthalmology*, Vol 10, No 4, 1914, pp 663-674.
102. Reveno, W.S.: "The Cause of Exophthalmic Goiter," *Archives of Internal Medicine*, Vol 48, Oct 1931, p 597.
103. Eustis, A.: "Some Interesting Observations on Goiter," *New Orleans Medical and Science Journal*, Vol 85, June 1933, pp 892-898.
104. Lane, W.A.: "Chronic Intestinal Stasis," *Journal of Surgery, Gynecology and Obstetrics*, Vol 16, 1913, p 602.
105. Von Noorden, C.: "Intoxication Proceeding From the Intestine, Especially Polyneuritis," *Journal of the American Medical Association*, Vol 60, No 2, 1913, p 104.
106. Von Noorden, *ibid*, p 105.
107. Herter, C.A. and Smith, E.E.: "Researches upon the Etiology of Idiopathic Epilepsy," *NY Medical Journal*, Vol 56, 1892, pp 208-211, 234-239, 260-266.
108. Satterlee, G.R. and Eldridge, W.W.: "Symptomatology of the Nervous System in Chronic Intestinal Toxemia," *Journal of the American Medical Association*, Vol 69, No 17, 1917, pp 1414-1418.
109. Haubold, *op cit*, pp 857-861.

110. Satterlee, *op cit*, p 1414.
111. Satterlee, *ibid*, p 1417.
112. Bainbridge, *op cit*, pp 437-443.
113. Nascher, I.L.: "Lane's Autointoxication Complex and the Manifestations of Senility," *NY Medical Journal*, Vol 100, No 6, 1914, p 256.
114. Osgood, R.B.: "Etiologic Factors in Certain Cases of So-Called Sciatic Scoliosis," *Journal of Bone and Joint Surgery*, Vol 9, Oct 1927, pp 667-676.
115. Von Noorden, *op cit*, p 103.
116. Schwartz, H.J.: "Association of Intestinal Indigestion with Various Dermatoses," *Archives of Dermatology and Syphilology*, Vol 13, 1926, p 674.
117. Burgess, J.F.: "Endogenous Irritants as Factors in Eczema and in Other Dermatoses," *Archives of Dermatology and Syphilology*, Vol 16, No 2, 1927, p 139.
118. Galloway, J.: "Cutaneous Indications of Alimentary Toxaemia," *British Medical Journal*, Vol 1, April 19, 1913, pp 815-817.
119. Bartle, *op cit*, p 28.
120. Lane, W.A.: "Consequences and Treatment from a Surgical Point of View," *British Medical Journal*, Vol 1, March 15, 1913, p 547.
121. Lane, W.A.: "Chronic Intestinal Stasis," *Journal of Surgery, Gynecology and Obstetrics*, Vol 16, 1913, p 601.
122. Bainbridge, *op cit*, p 443.
123. Prehn, R.T.: "A Clonal Selection Theory of Chemical Carcinogenesis," *Journal of National Cancer Institute*, Vol 32, No 1, Jan 1964, p 1.
124. Satterlee, G.R.: "Autogenous Colon Vaccines in the Study, Diagnosis and Therapy of Chronic Intestinal Toxemia," *Journal of American Medical Association*, Vol 67, No 24, 1916, p 1731.
125. Bartle, *op cit*, p 448.
126. Goodhart, R.S. and Shils, M.E.: *Modern Nutrition in Health and Disease*, 5th ed, Lea and Febiger, Philadelphia, 1973, p 30.
127. Hegsted, D.M.: "Minimum Protein Requirements of Adults," *American Journal of Clinical Nutrition*, Vol 21, No 5, May 1968, pp 352-357.
128. Turck, F.B.: "Intestinal Venous Stasis: Diffusion of Bacteria and Other Colloids," *Boston Medical and Surgical Journal*, Vol 176, No 19, 1917, p 665.
129. Soper, H.W.: "Autointoxication in Chronic Constipation," *Journal of the American Medical Association*, Vol 69, No 18, 1917, p 1512.
130. Bartle, *op cit*, p 447.
131. Stucky, *op cit*, p 1186.
132. Synnott, *op cit*, p 444.
133. Saundby, R.: "Alimentary Toxemia: Its Symptoms and Treatment," *British Medical Journal*, Vol 1, March 15, 1913, p 545.
134. Dubin, *op cit*, p 91.
135. Gerard, R.W.: "The Lethal Agent in Acute Intestinal Obstruction," *Journal of American Medical Association*, Vol 79, No 19, 1922, p 1583.
136. Sherwin, C.P. and Hawk, P.B.: "Fasting Studies: VII. The Putrefaction Processes in the Intestine of a Man During Fasting and During Subsequent Periods of Low and High Protein Ingestion," *Journal of Biological Chemistry*, Vol 11, No 3, 1912, p 177.
137. Fitch, W.E.: "Putrefactive Intestinal Toxemia," *Medical Journal and Record*, Vol 132, Aug 20, 1930, p 186.
138. Bainbridge, *op cit*, p 440.
139. Soper, H.W.: "Autointoxication in Chronic Constipation," *Journal of the American Medical Association*, Vol 69, No 18, 1917, p 1512.
140. Bassler, A.: "Chronic Intestinal Toxemia," *Medical Record*, Vol 145, 1937, p 159.
141. Fordtran, J.S., Scroggie, W.B., and Polter, D.E.: "Colonic absorption of tryptophan metabolites in man," *J Lab and Clin Med*, Vol 64, 1964, p 125-132.
142. Bakke, O.M.: "Urinary simple phenols in rats fed purified and nonpurified diets," *J Nutr*, Vol 98, 1969, p 209.
143. Folin, *op cit*, p 309.
144. Bakke, O.M.: "Urinary simple phenols in rats fed diets containing different amounts of casein and 10% tyrosine," *J Nutr*, Vol 98, 1969, pp 217-221.
145. Aarbakke, J. and Schjönsby, H.: "Value of urinary simple phenol and indican determinations in the diagnosis of the stagnant loop syndrome," *Scand J Gastroent*, Vol 11, 1976, pp 409-414.
146. Tomkin, G.H. and Weir, D.G.: *Quart J Med*, Vol 41, 1972, pp 191-203.
147. Fordtran, et al, *op cit*.
148. Neale, G., Lambert, R.A., and Gorbach, S.L.: "The production of indole by bacteria in **vitro**," *Gut*, Vol 10, 1969, pp 1056-1057.
149. Happold, F.C.: "Tryptophanase-tryptophan reaction," *Advances in Enzymology*, Vol 10, 1950, p 51.
150. Donaldson, R.M., Jr.: "Malabsorption of Co^{60}-Labeled Cyanocobalamin in Rats with Intestinal Diverticula. 1. Evaluation of Possible Mechanisms," *Gastroenterology*, Vol 43, 1962, p 271.
151. Robbins, *op cit*, p 55.
152. Thorn, G.W., Adams, R.D., Bruanwald, E., Isselbacher, K.J., Petersdorf, R.G.: *Harrison's Principles of Internal Medicine*, 8th ed, McGraw-Hill Book Co, New York, NY, 1977, p 715.
153. Thorn, *ibid*, p 1606.
154. Thorn, *ibid*, p 1909.
155. Tabaqchali, S., *Scand J Gastroent*. 1970 Suppl, Vol 6, pp 139-163.
156. Bakke, O.M., *Scand J Gastroent*, Vol 4, 1969, pp 603-608.
157. Alam, S.Q., Boctor, A.M., Rogers, Q.R., and Harper, A.E.: "Some effects of amino acids and cortisol on tyrosine toxicity in the rat," *J Nutr*, Vol 93, 1967, p 317.
158. Bakke, O.M.: "Urinary simple phenols in rats fed diets containing different amounts of casein and 10% tyrosine," *J Nutr*, Vol 98, 1969, pp 217-221.
159. Horning, E.C., and Dalgliesh, C.E.: "The association of skatole-forming bacteria in the small intestine with the malabsorption syndrome and certain anemias," *Biochem J*, Vol 70, 1958, p 13.
160. Izquierdo, J.A., and Stoppani, A.D.M.: "Inhibition of smooth muscle contractility by indole and some indole compounds," *Brit J Pharmacol*, Vol 8, 1953, pp 389-394.
161. Proctor, M.H.: "Bacterial dissimilation of indoleacetic acid: a new route of breakdown of the indole nucleus," *Nature*, Vol 181, 1958, p 1345.
162. Horning, E.C. and Dalgliesh, C.E.: "The association of skatole-forming bacteria in the small intestine with the malabsorption syndrome and certain anemias," *Biochemical J*, Vol 70, 1958, p 13.
163. Sprince, H.: "Biochemical aspects of indole metabolism in normal and schizophrenic subjects," *Annals New York Academy of Sciences*, Vol 96, 1962, pp 399-418.
164. Dalgliesch, C.E., Kelly, W., and Horning, E.C.: "Excretion of a sulphatoxy derivative of skatole in pathological states in man," *Biochemical J*, Vol 70, 1958, p 13.
165. Horning, E.C., Sweeley, C.C., and Kelly, W.: "Mammalian hydroxylation in the 6-position of the indole ring," *Biochem Biophys Acta*, Vol 32, 1959, pp 566-567.

Appendix - H: Tesla Lightwear Sunglasses

Tesla Lightwear Optics

Light is the ultimate form of all electromagnetic energy. Light has dual wave-particle nature that has been revealed in quantum mechanics. This duality is shared by all primary constituents of nature. Through evolution, we became adapted to diffused sunlight, which includes high energy UV and a high-energy visible light (called blue-violet light from 380 to 450 nm) which keeps us on constant alert.

BIOPTRON has developed a method for transforming the light into a more beneficial form of light. Based on our patented technology and initial scientific pilot studies we recommend wearing the Tesla HyperLight Optics as a replacement for sunglasses, for blocking UV and highly energetic blue sunlight, as well as for possible relaxing effect, improved decision-making processes, and protection against the harmful portion of blue-violet light emitted by LCD and LED screens (as replacement for blue blocker glasses).

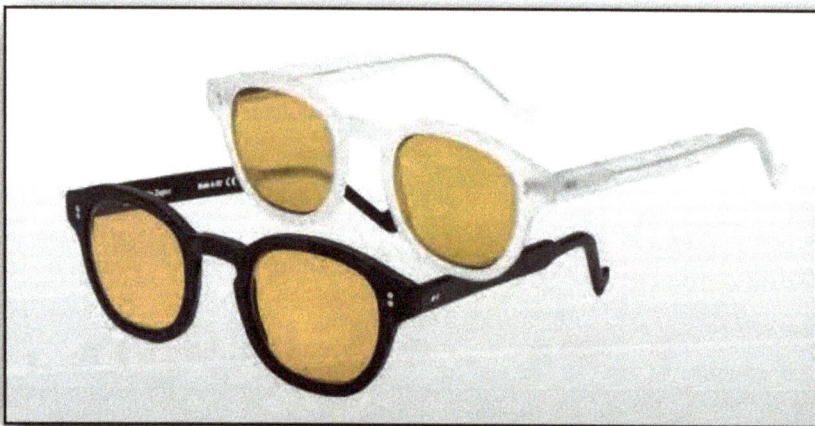

We spend today more than 60% of our time in front of computer screens and phone screens. When the artificial LED white light or LED from mobile devices and computers passes through the Tesla HyperLight Optics, it gets shifted into a light spectrum away from the harmful UV and blue-violet light and becomes hyperharmonized at the same time. The light spectrum of Tesla HyperLight Optics corresponds perfectly with the eye sensibility spectrum.

Tesla Lightwear Optics

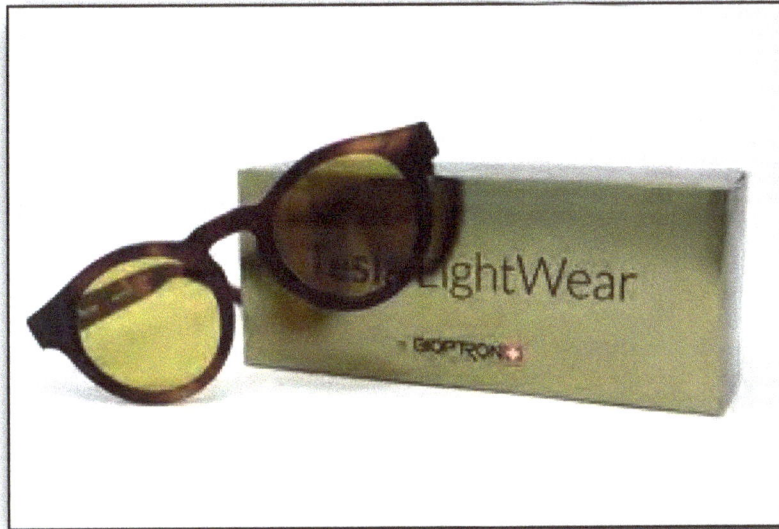

Quantum Healing with Hyperpolarized Sunglasses
by Gerald H. Smith, DDS, IMD

The use of light for healing is not a new concept. However, the use of hyperpolarized sunglasses as a new healing modality provides healthcare practitioners with an innovative technology that has great healing potential. The Swiss company, Zepter, has pioneered the use of man-made full-spectrum light for enhancing the body's ability to restore homeostasis. A recent clinical observation has spawned a new paradigm for patient treatment.

Since the human body functions within a normal frequency ranging from 62 to 68 MHz, any alteration that lowers the frequency range transitions the body into the disease process. It has been documented that disease starts at 58 MHz with the appearance of colds and flu at 57 to 60 MHz, Epstein-Barr virus occurs at 55 MHz, cancer initiates at 42 MHz, and death starts at 25 MHz. Elevating the body's frequency level by means of raw organic foods, homeopathic remedies, food based vitamins, minerals, scalar waves, essential oils, prayer and meditation, music, sunlight, Rife frequencies, and color light therapy all function to restore health.

Tesla Lightwear Optics

In the 1970s, a German researcher by the name of Fritz Albert Popp discovered that carcinogens, like mercury, prevent the body from absorbing the wavelength of 280 nm to repair the DNA. This process triggers degeneration and disease. This blocking effect holds true for all carcinogens and prevents the DNA repair process.

Fortuitously, this researcher recently discovered that placing the Tesla Lightwear glasses on someone who had a toxic substance like mercury in her pocket negates the deleterious effect of the mercury. The subject was tested kinesiologically to establish a baseline response. The muscles tested strong. Then a vial of mercury was placed in the subject's pocket, and she was retested. The retest resulted in the subject not being able to hold up her arms. The Tesla Lightwear glasses were then placed over her eyes while the vial of mercury was still in her pocket, and the subject tested stronger than had been on the baseline test. My hypothesis is that the frequency generated by the vial of mercury disrupted the subject's energetic field. Placement of the Tesla Lightwear glasses stimulated the central and peripheral nervous systems, via the optic nerve, with full-spectrum light (430–770 THz - minus the infrared and blue portions) to raise the energy field of the entire body from the inside outward. I believe this higher frequency has the beneficial effect of negating the 13 to 20 toxic frequencies that mercury produces. Extrapolating this finding, my theory is that wearing the Tesla Lightwear glasses will neutralize all toxic energy fields from pesticides, chemicals, heavy metals, vaccines, viruses, etc. by raising the frequency level of the body's energy field. In essence, the full-spectrum light will either transmutate toxic energy fields into nontoxic energy or erase them. Further study is needed to confirm these observations.

The Tesla Lightwear Sunglasses can be ordered directly from the North American division of Zepter International by calling (647) 748-1115.

www.ingramcontent.com/pod-product-compliance
Lightning Source LLC
Chambersburg PA
CBHW042338030426
42335CB00030B/3386